WHAT OTHERS ARE SAYING ABOUT
FIT FOR THE KING:

"*Fit for the King* is an inspiring and motivational weight loss guide. The scriptural basis for his book provides people of faith with a clear understanding that God is truly concerned about us taking care of our bodies through good nutrition and physical activity. Through this book, I believe Thomas Hundley will inspire many people on the road toward improving their spiritual and physical health."

—*Reverend Jeannette Jordan*
registered dietitian and certified Diabetes educator
owner, J & J Health Consultants
president, the Minority Heath Education Network

"I lost sixteen pounds in forty days without any effort at all. This book is the simplest program you will ever follow."

—*Kellie Starling*, Lugoff, South Carolina

"After week three, my cholesterol had dropped one hundred points. I am now able to walk every day without pain in my joints and legs."

—*James Joseph Scott*, Atlanta, Georgia

"This book is a motivator because it will enhance your confidence and help you to understand the importance of being healthy."

—*Judy Warren*, Harrisburg, North Carolina

"I squeezed into a size fourteen when I started; now I'm a comfortable size twelve."

—*Ericka Burrus-Moore*, Columbia, South Carolina

"I am sixty years old with high blood pressure and type 2 diabetes. Not only is this a good diet, but it's also helping me to eat right."

—*Shirley Palmer*, Columbia, South Carolina

"This book has helped me to understand that God made me to be a big girl, but He demands that I be healthy. I lost twenty-two pounds after week five."

—*Donnie Johnson*, Tacoma, Washington

"To my amazement, I have lost thirteen pounds. What?! I knew this program was working; I knew it was like no other. But thirteen pounds? What a boost!"

—*Andrea Brazil*, Eastover, South Carolina

"I love the way this book is designed, especially the inspirational thoughts along with Scripture, which help to put things into perspective."

—*John Loper*, Waynesboro, Mississippi

"This book has changed my life. The amazing thing is that it is so simple. I love the one-day-at-time approach."

—*Kathleen Nurse,* Columbia, South Carolina

"I have been on blood pressure medication for more than six years. As of yesterday, I had lost twenty-two pounds, and my doctor now says that I no longer have to take my medicine. Glory hallelujah!"

—*Rhonda Jordan*, Millington, Tennessee

FIT FOR**THE KING**

THOMAS**HUNDLEY**

FIT FOR**THE KING**

GOD'S PLAN FOR WEIGHT LOSS AND TOTAL HEALTH

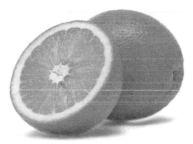

ω
WHITAKER
HOUSE

No liability is assumed with respect to the use of the information contained within. Although every precaution has been taken, neither Whitaker House nor Thomas L. Hundley assumes liability for any errors or omissions. Neither is any liability assumed for damages resulting from the use of the information contained herein. It is recommended that you always consult your health care professional before beginning this or any other health and fitness program.

FIT FOR THE KING
God's Plan for Weight Loss and Total Health
(with workout DVD included)

Thomas L. Hundley
info@fitforakingfitness.com
www.fitforakingfitness.com

Fit for a King Fitness
P.O. Box 29406
Charlotte, NC 28229

ISBN: 978-1-60374-078-4
Printed in the United States of America
© 2009 by Thomas L. Hundley

Whitaker House
1030 Hunt Valley Circle
New Kensington, PA 15068
www.whitakerhouse.com

Library of Congress Cataloging-in-Publication Data

Hundley, Thomas, 1972–
 Fit for the king / Thomas Hundley.
   p. cm.
Includes bibliographical references.
 Summary: "A 40-day, Bible-based guide to diet, fitness, and spiritual growth designed to encourage people into the shape that God meant for them to be"—Provided by publisher.
 ISBN 978-1-60374-078-4 (trade pbk. w/ dvd : alk. paper) 1. Physical fitness—Religious aspects—Christianity. 2. Health—Religious aspects—Christianity. 3. Spiritual formation. I. Title.

 BV4598.H86 2009
 248.4—dc22

                                         2008040287

    2 3 4 5 6 7 8 9 10 11 12 **UI** 17 16 15 14 13 12 11 10 09

DEDICATION

This book is dedicated to six women in my life who have served to make me the man that I am today.

First, to my late great-grandmother, Mrs. Ordella Jordan, who used her gift of prophecy to tell me that God was going to use me to touch the world.

To my grandmother, Bethel Hundley, who has always made me feel as though I was the chosen one.

To my mother, Fannie L. Gray, whose loving sacrifices and guidance provided me the means and the way to pursue my dreams.

To my daughters, Peyton and Erin, who serve as my reasons and my inspirations for living an exemplary life.

And, most importantly, to the one whom God placed on this earth just for me—my wife, Amy—whose love and support serve as the wind beneath my wings.

ACKNOWLEDGMENTS

I would like to extend a special word of thanks to Mr. Johnny Loper, certified sports nutritionist, personal trainer, and owner of Jay Lo Fitness Personal Training Studio, for his joint collaboration in developing the safe and effective meal plan presented in this book. Our meal plan is the product of two years of extensive research and testing. Mr. Loper and I sincerely believe that individuals are more likely to remain committed to eating properly if provided with a structured and flexible plan. We also believe that an individual's commitment is further enhanced when he or she is provided with a variety of healthy foods that he or she routinely purchases. The meal plan within this book is centered on those beliefs and will serve as the cornerstone of your healthier lifestyle. Thanks, Jay Lo, for your knowledge, expertise, and friendship.

To learn more about Johnny and his fitness studio, visit www.jaylofitness.com.

CONTENTS

PREFACE

G od is using me as His instrument of choice to deliver a very important message. This message, which has become this book, is not intended to frighten but rather to inform and educate all who struggle with obesity or being overweight. It is also intended to help those who suffer because of unhealthy eating habits, sedentary lifestyles, and poor health. This message should not be taken lightly or put off until some later date. For some of you, this may be your final opportunity to make the necessary changes to improve your health. The fact that you are reading this book is no coincidence. God loves you so much that He has personally sent you another opportunity to receive the blessings He intends for you to enjoy.

I believe that God's message to you is this: "My dear child, I have stated in My Word that you shall place no other gods before Me. I have provided you with many earthly things, but you have not used those things in a manner that brings glory to My kingdom. You have not treated your body as a temple of the Holy Spirit. You must present yourself as one approved. Show yourself faithful in the small matters that I place before you. When you are able to do this, I will bless you with even greater things. You must present your body to Me as a living sacrifice so that it may bring honor and glory to the kingdom of heaven."

Fit for the King may be God's way of giving you another opportunity to be faithful and obedient. You must not place food or laziness before God. The Lord is asking for forty days of obedience—your opportunity to finally lose weight, get in shape, and improve your health. And it begins today!

Introduction

What size are you supposed to be? Hollywood's answer to that question seems to be, "Slim, trim, and no larger than a size two." Your parents' answer to that question might be "thick, curvaceous, and anywhere below a size twenty." Your friends' answer to that question might be, "You look fine just the way you are." In truth, there is only one Person qualified to answer that question. It is not your doctor, your dietician, or your personal trainer. The answer to that question is best answered by the One who created you—God!

Before you were born, God planned for you to be a certain size and shape. He intended for you to be capable of maintaining that size and shape without major dietary restrictions and without laborious physical effort. You are probably thinking, *This sounds too good to be true. Why haven't I heard about this before?* With God's help, you will discover *your* perfect size and shape.

Do you think that God intended for every living person to be the same size and shape? Do you think He had a cookie-cutter design for his human assembly line? I don't think so. The same God who made Shaquille O'Neal also made Michael J. Fox. The same God who made Queen Latifah also made Sarah Jessica Parker. It is humanly impossible for Shaq to ever look like Michael J., just as it is humanly unnatural for Latifah to ever look like Sarah Jessica. God made each one of these special people to have and maintain his or her unique size and shape. Likewise, you were made by the same God to have your own special size and shape.

You may have participated in diets or programs that required you to do some crazy things: cut carbohydrates; eat nothing but grapefruit; eat only prepackaged foods; never eat desserts; or never eat red meat. I believe the Lord's response to those man-made methods and ideologies would be something like this: "My children, I have created everything on earth for your enjoyment. I have provided you with many different foods to eat and drink. Everything I have created is My gift to you. You now have a choice how to care for the things I have provided. I have written in My Word that it is a sin to be gluttonous. Moderation and order are pleasing in My eyes. Show yourselves worthy of even greater gifts."

If you been living a gluttonous lifestyle and eating self-indulgently, you probably are not the size and shape God intended you to be. Don't worry! As many others have found out, in your hands you are now holding the solution to your problems.

It is an amazing honor to be chosen by God to carry out His works. While writing this book, I have established a closer and more personal relationship with Him. I have developed an understanding of His Word and an appreciation for His magnificence that surpasses my wildest imagination. Over the past five months, it was almost as if my fingers were on the computer keyboard but I was not in control of what I was typing. That is how I feel sure that this book is going to change and save the lives of many people who have struggled to lose weight and combat obesity. I can think of few missions as fulfilling as helping you to live a healthier, longer, and happier life. The Lord has prepared me for a mission, He has given me the message, and He has demanded that I share it with the world.

Today, I want you to open your hearts and minds to receive the Word of the Lord as it relates to diet, nutrition, health, and fitness. When you finally reach your predetermined size and shape, you will realize that your overall health is better, your energy level is higher, and your diet is less restrictive.

Every journey begins with a step, and every step has a direction. The Bible states, *"A man's heart plans his way, but the LORD directs his steps"* (Proverbs 16:9 NKJV). By choosing to read this book, you have placed your feet firmly on the path that leads to God's answer to your problems. Your first step begins today!

> *I will instruct you and teach you in the way you should go; I will counsel you and watch over you.*
>
> (Psalm 32:8)

Your Daily Bread

For the next forty days and forty nights, you will take a journey that will transform your body, improve your health, and change your life. This book is divided into forty brief chapters, each representing a different step of spiritual, physical, and nutritional growth. Each chapter will take less than ten minutes to read, but you *must* read, consume, and digest each chapter one day at a time. Each chapter contains five sections that I call the Five Loaves of Bread:

- **Bread for the Mind.** This section is equivalent to your one-a-day vitamin. Just as your body needs a balanced intake of nutrients for optimal performance, your mind needs a balanced intake of teaching and wisdom. As you take each daily step on this journey, this section will provide you with daily "food for thought" to ponder along the way.

- **Bread for the Spirit.** This section will lead you to the "bread of heaven" mentioned in the Bible. (See Psalm 105:40.) You will be given a Bible verse to read, along with a brief devotional thought to ponder.

- **Bread for the Soul.** This section contains a brief daily prayer to help facilitate one-on-one conversations with God. This is your opportunity to communicate with God through prayer and reflection. It also provides a section where you can journal your thoughts, prayers, and experiences.

- **Bread for the Body.** This section provides you with your recommended daily physical fitness regimen. Feel free to use your own favorite exercises, workout routine, or fitness program. I have included a workout DVD from my own organization, Fit For a King Fitness Ministries. This aerobics video is designed to target, tone, and tighten your body while providing a daily mix of aerobic and anaerobic activity. It also provides additional spiritual insights to jump-start your day.

- **Bread for the Day.** This section serves as your daily nourishment and sustenance. It provides you with a structured plan to help you eat a balanced diet, as the Lord intends you to. This section details what to eat, when to eat, how much to eat, and how often to eat for the next forty days. It also provides a section where you can journal your food choices. Refer to the Food Exchange List at the back of the book to substitute food choices that appeal to your own taste and lifestyle.

I have often asked myself, *Why did the Lord choose me for this mission?* Let's face it: there is no shortage of fitness professionals who are qualified, certified, and experienced in helping people lose weight. God answered my question by directing my attention to 1 Samuel 17—the story of David and Goliath. Like David, I am here to defeat a giant problem. David went to battle against Goliath; I am going to battle obesity. I face this giant not as an armed soldier but as an armed servant. David defeated his giant with a sling, five smooth stones, and a sword. This book represents my sling, the Five Loaves of Bread represent my five stones, and the Bible represents my sword. My prayer is that, like David, I was chosen because I am the right man for the job.

As I read the story of David and Goliath, I am fascinated by the descriptive similarities, especially the part that says

David was young, ruddy, and good-looking. (See 1 Samuel 17:42.) I guess it goes without saying that David was also very confident. As you read the story for yourself, you will find that David had an army behind him. *You* represent the army. Together, with God's help, we will achieve our victory by defeating our modern-day giant. Let's go to work!

Do you not know that your body is the temple of the Holy Spirit, who is in you, whom you have received from God? You are not your own; you were bought at a price. Therefore honor God with your body.

(1 Corinthians 6:19–20)

THE CONTRACT

I, ___Susan Martinez___ (your name), do solemnly affirm that from this day, _____, (today's date), I will become a better steward of the Lord's possessions. I *commit* to living and maintaining a healthier lifestyle through proper nutrition and physical fitness using God's methods. I *accept* that the Lord has placed me on this path, but it is I who must choose the direction. I *acknowledge* that the Lord will order my steps, but I must decide to move my feet. I *understand* that the only way for me to achieve my goals is to center my life on the plan the Lord has for me and not the plan I have for myself. Finally, I agree to take this forty-day journey along this Christ-centered path toward spiritual, nutritional, and physical improvement. This is the signed covenant of my decision to "let go and let God!"

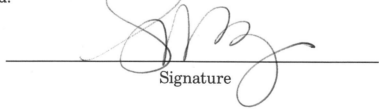

_____
Signature

For where two or three come together in my name, there am I with them. (Matthew 18:20)

The words in this passage of Scripture represent Christ's promise to you. Fitness is a lot like life in that we sometimes need a spotter, a partner, a coach, or a teammate to help us along the way. I encourage you to find a partner to assist you along this journey.

Partner's Name

Though one may be overpowered, two can defend themselves. A cord of three strands is not quickly broken. (Ecclesiastes 4:12)

Your Beginning Fitness Profile

This is your book; write in it, tab it, and highlight your favorite passages in it. Let it serve as your personal, nutritional and spiritual journal for the next forty days. I want you to journal your personal thoughts, struggles, temptations, victories, defeats, ups, downs, disappointments, and achievements. Your first entry will be a record of your personal information. Exactly forty days from the date you start, you will use the information below to compare the *old* you to the *new* you. The ultimate purpose of this record is to document the power and the greatness of God.

Date: _____

Name: _____

Height: ____ft._____in.   Weight: _____lbs.

Neck: _____in.   Chest: _____in.

Waist: _____in.   Hips: _____in.

Body fat percentage: _____
http://www.bmi-calculator.net/body-fat-calculator/

Dress or pant size:_____

Blood pressure: _____

Cholesterol level: _____

These last two are best done by visiting a physician—something you should do whenever starting a diet or exercise program.

THE OLD YOU

— Your photo here —

You, dear children, are from God and have overcome them, because the one who is in you is greater than the one who is in the world. (1 John 4:4)

THE TEN COMMANDMENTS OF CHRISTIAN WEIGHT LOSS

Through extensive research and devoted prayer, I received from the Lord a nutritional guide designed to help you shed pounds and inches while improving your overall health. When your forty-day journey is complete, you will rejoice in the miracles of your weight loss. You will marvel at the sight of your new body. The Lord will also reveal to you what size He wants you to keep for the rest of your life. There are rules to follow as you take this journey. I call them the Ten Commandments of Christian Weight Loss.

The Ten Commandments of Christian Weight Loss

1. Thou shalt drink *only* water for forty days.
2. Thou shalt begin *every* day with prayer.
3. Thou shalt not consume *any* fried food for forty days.
4. Thou shalt not use *any* table salt or seasoning salt for forty days.
5. Thou shalt drink *at least* 64 ounces of water each day.
6. Thou shalt consume *only* fruits or vegetables after 8:00 p.m.
7. Thou shalt pack your lunch and snacks *daily* to avoid eating out.
8. Thou shalt keep a daily journey to record *all* foods consumed each day.
9. Thou shalt substitute *only* the foods recommended on the Food Exchange List.
10. Thou shalt weigh yourself *only* on the days recommended by this book.

This calls for patient endurance on the part of the saints who obey God's commandments and remain faithful to Jesus. (Revelation 14:12)

Food Choices and Preparation

- Use a low-fat dressing (condiment) of choice for salads, sandwiches, and dipped vegetables. Examples include light mayonnaise, light ranch dressing, vinaigrette dressings, and mustard.

- Use whole grain breads instead of white breads for sandwiches.

- Use herbs and spices rather than salt to add flavor to meals without loading up on sodium.

- Prepare all meats in whatever way you desire but avoid deep frying or using heavy cooking oils. Coconut oil is the best option because it is low in saturated fat and has a high smoking point.

- Use fresh vegetables whenever possible; frozen are also acceptable. Steaming vegetables is always a healthy method of preparation.

For God did not give us a spirit of timidity, but a spirit of power, of love and of self-discipline.
(2 Timothy 1:7)

Week 1

You Gotta Choose a Path!

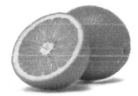

TESTIMONIALS

"I lost sixteen pounds in forty days without any effort at all. This book is the simplest program you will ever follow. I actually lost ten pounds within the first three weeks without ever exercising. The Food Exchange List in the back is a godsend. After the first week, I figured out what foods were going to work for me and stuck with them. I would recommend this program to anyone who wants to lose weight while getting closer to God. This is the last diet plan you will ever need."

—Kellie Starling, Lugoff, South Carolina

"God is so good. This book must have been sent directly from heaven. I am forty-three years old, and before I read this book I was badly out of shape. After week three, my cholesterol had dropped one hundred points. I am now able to walk every day without pain in my joints and legs. But the best thing that happened to me from this book is that I have started reading the Bible every day. I know that the Lord is smiling on me."

—James Joseph Scott, Atlanta, Georgia

WEEK 1 SHOPPING LIST

List represents meal plan choices and alternatives:

Fresh Vegetables	Fresh Fruits	Canned/ Frozen	Meat	Seafood
17 servings Choose your favorites: • Asparagus • Broccoli • Carrots • Cauliflower • Celery • Cucumbers • Green beans • Lettuce • Onions • Peppers • Potatoes • Spinach • Sprouts • Squash • Tomatoes • Zucchini Other:	14 servings Choose your favorites: • Apples • Bananas • Blueberries • Cherries • Grapes • Kiwis • Lemons • Limes • Melons • Oranges • Peaches • Pears • Plums • Raspberries • Strawberries • Tangerines Other:	• Peas • Mixed veggies • Pickles • Pineapple • Vegetable soup • Tomato soup • Tuna Substitutes: • Applesauce • Beans • Beets • Mixed fruit • Olives	• 5 chicken breasts • Ground turkey • Lunch meat • Turkey bacon • Turkey breast • Turkey sausage Other:	3 servings Choose your favorites: • Crab • Flounder • Halibut • Salmon • Sardines • Scallops • Tilapia • Trout • Tuna steak Other:

Misc. Groceries	Cereal	Dairy	Breads	Snacks
• Coleslaw • Honey • Jelly/Jam • Reduced fat mayonnaise • Natural peanut butter • Potato salad • White rice • Wild rice • Salad dressings (low-fat) Other:	7 servings Choose your favorites: Cold: • All-Bran • Cheerios • Grape Nuts • Life • Raisin Bran • Shredded Wheat • Granola • Special K Hot: • Cream of wheat • Kasha • Oatmeal Other:	• Eggs • Milk (1% or skim) • Sour cream • Yogurt Other:	• Bagels • Buns • English muffins • Whole grain bread Alternatives: • Crackers • Pita bread • Rolls • Spinach wraps • Wheat wraps	• Almonds • Granola bars • Popcorn • Pretzel rods • Raisins • Salsa Substitutes: • Cashews • Creamsicles • Dried fruit • Multigrain chips • Oatmeal cookies • Special K bars

ACCEPTANCE

Step 1

BREAD FOR THE MIND

Congratulations! You have chosen to follow God's path to weight loss and physical fitness. Now that you have chosen your path, the Lord will order your steps. Your first step is to **accept** certain facts of life. We will define *acceptance* as "the act of wholeheartedly welcoming and receiving." Here are the things that God wants you to accept:

- ***Accept* the fact that God made you and knows you inside and out.**

  For you created my inmost being; you knit me together in my mother's womb. (Psalm 139:13)

- ***Accept* the fact that you need God's help.**

  Even when you are old, I will be the same. Even when your hair has turned gray, I will take care of you.

  (Isaiah 46:4 NCV)

- ***Accept* the fact that your way has failed.**

  I have labored to no purpose; I have spent my strength in vain and for nothing. (Isaiah 49:4)

- ***Accept* the Bible as your daily moral authority.**

  All Scripture is inspired by God and is useful for teaching, for showing people what is wrong in their lives, for correcting faults, and for teaching how to live right. (2 Timothy 3:16 NCV)

- ***Accept* the help that God is giving you through this book.**

  Let this be written for a future generation, that a people not yet created may praise the LORD.

  (Psalm 102:18)

BREAD FOR THE SPIRIT
(Read Romans 8:5–9)

Accept the fact that God wants to free you from your situation. He wants to bless you with the desires of your heart. First, however, you must prove to Him that you are obedient. He knows that your struggles with gluttony, temptation, flesh, and other things keep you from giving Him your all. You must acknowledge and understand God's role in your life. He made you and He knows exactly what it will take to save you. Accept these facts today! By accepting these facts, your first step is pointed in the direction of victory. From this day forward, we will take *one* step at a time, *one* day at a time, and *one* meal at a time.

They that are in the flesh cannot please GOD. (v8)

BREAD FOR THE SOUL

The steps of a good man are ordered by the LORD, and He delights in his way. (Psalm 37:23 NKJV)

Say this prayer and write down any thoughts or requests you have for God:

Father, as I take my first steps on the road to physical and spiritual fitness, I pray that You will order my steps. I thank You for bringing me to this point in my life. I accept the fact that my way has failed and I sincerely need Your help. I pray that You will continue to guide and direct my path today and always. Amen.

_____

_____

_____

_____

_____

_____

_____

_____

_____

_____

_____

BREAD FOR THE BODY

Perform thirty minutes of cardiorespiratory and/or aerobic activity.

Day 1	Exercise Options	What I Did
30 minutes	Walk	
	Run	
	Treadmill	
	Aerobics	
	Elliptical	
	Bicycle	
	Fit for the King DVD	

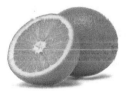

8/4/09

BREAD FOR THE DAY

Day 1	What to Eat	What I Ate
Breakfast	1 cup cereal	
6:30–7:30 a.m.	6 oz. low-fat milk	
	2 slices turkey bacon	
	1 apple	
Mid-morning Snack	1 granola bar	
9:30–10:00 a.m.	1 pear	
Lunch	4 oz. turkey sandwich w/lettuce and tomato	
12:00–1:00 p.m.	1 cup vegetable soup	
Mid-afternoon Snack	½ English muffin	
3:00–3:30 p.m.	1 Tbsp. jelly	
Dinner	4 oz. grilled chicken	
5:30–8:00 p.m.	½ cup wild rice	
	1 cup green beans	
Calories	**1400–1800**	

CHANGE

Step 2

BREAD FOR THE MIND

Your next step in the Christian weight loss process is to undergo **change**. There are many definitions for the word *change*, but we are going to use the definition that refers to *repentance*, "the act of turning around and going in another direction." You must change from going *your* way and begin going *God's* way instead:

- **Change the way you think.**

  Do not conform any longer to the pattern of this world, but be transformed by the renewing of your mind. Then you will be able to test and approve what God's will is—his good, pleasing and perfect will.

  (Romans 12:2)

- **Change the way you see.**

  But one thing I do: forgetting what is behind and straining toward what is ahead, I press on toward the goal. (Philippians 3:13–14)

- **Change the way you act.**

  Blessed is the man who does not walk in the counsel of the wicked or stand in the way of sinners or sit in the seat of mockers. (Psalm 1:1)

- **Change the way you eat.**

  When your words came, I ate them; they were my joy and my heart's delight, for I bear your name, O LORD God Almighty. (Jeremiah 15:16)

BREAD FOR THE SPIRIT
(Read Ephesians 4:22–24)

Change is good because God is good. If you have been traveling along the same road and it continues to lead you to dead ends, at some point you will need to consider changing your route. The same logic applies in your efforts to lose weight. To achieve the miraculous and permanent results that you desire, you must change from "man's" way of thinking to "God's" way of thinking. Once you start traveling in God's direction, your repentance, or change, means that you intend never to return to your old ways. This change leads you down the road to salvation, and the road to salvation leads you to the land of promised miracles. Are you ready for your miracle?

*put off the old man —
put on the new man!*

BREAD FOR THE SOUL

"For I know the plans I have for you," declares the LORD, "plans to prosper you and not to harm you, plans to give you hope and a future."

(Jeremiah 29:11)

Say this prayer and write down any thoughts or requests you have for God:

Father, I realize that my way has failed. Lord, open my eyes to accept and understand the changes that I need to make in my life. I pray that You will help me to understand Your plan for me. Your plan is amazing and I place my trust and hope in You. Amen.

BREAD FOR THE BODY

Perform thirty minutes of aerobic and anaerobic exercise today. Your workout session should target toning your lower body with emphasis on the thighs, hips, and buttocks.

Day 2	Exercise Options	What I Did
30 minutes	Free weights	
	Strength training	
	Aerobics	
	Dumbbells	
	Resistance training	
	Fit for the King DVD	

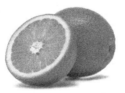

8|5|09

BREAD FOR THE DAY

Day 2	What to Eat	What I Ate
Breakfast	1 cup cereal	
6:30–7:30 a.m.	6 oz. low-fat milk	
	½ cup raisins	
	1 slice toast w/ 1 Tbsp. jelly/jam	
Mid-morning Snack	1 granola bar	
9:30–10:00 a.m.	1 banana	
Lunch	A 4-oz. grilled chicken sub w/ lettuce and tomato	
12:00–1:00 p.m.	1 cup tomato soup	
Mid-afternoon Snack	¼ cup almonds	
3:00–3:30 p.m.	6 strawberries	
Dinner	6 oz. baked fish	
5:30–8:00 p.m.	1 cup broccoli	
	1 baked potato	
	2 Tbsp. salsa	
Calories	**1500–1800**	

Step 3

BREAD FOR THE MIND

This is the most fulfilling step that you will take on your journey. You could actually remain frozen in this step for days and still not learn all you need to know. This step is so important that I have provided two biblical references for each point. It would take me more than one hundred pages to accurately define **love**, and still I would probably miss the mark. My definition of *love* is "the uncontrollable and unconditional feelings of joy and pain, happiness and sadness, and calm and chaos that one feels for another." For today, we will use God's definition of love: "the unconditional regard and highest esteem held for all of God's children." Today, we will learn to *love*.

- **Love God.**

  Love the LORD your God with all your heart and with all your soul and with all your strength.

  (Deuteronomy 6:5)

  Jesus replied: "Love the Lord your God with all your heart and with all your soul and with all your mind." This is the first and greatest commandment.

  (Matthew 22:37–38)

- **Love yourself.**

  The Father himself loves you because you have loved me and have believed that I came from God.
  (John 16:27)

  If I give all I possess to the poor and surrender my body to the flames, but have not love, I gain nothing.
  (1 Corinthians 13:3)

- **Love your neighbor.**

  The entire law is summed up in a single command: "Love your neighbor as yourself."
  (Galatians 5:14)

  And he has given us this command: Whoever loves God must also love his brother.
  (1 John 4:21)

- **Love your enemies.**

  This is love: not that we loved God, but that he loved us and sent his Son as an atoning sacrifice for our sins. Dear friends, since God so loved us, we also ought to love one another.
  (1 John 4:10–11)

  Finally, all of you, live in harmony with one another; be sympathetic, love as brothers, be compassionate and humble.
  (1 Peter 3:8–9)

- **Love as a way of life.**

  This is love: that we walk in obedience to his commands. As you have heard from the beginning, his command is that you walk in love.
  (2 John 1:6)

  Follow the way of love.
  (1 Corinthians 14:1)

BREAD FOR THE SPIRIT
(Read 1 Corinthians 13)

Love lasts forever and conquers all. There is no greater earthly force than love. Whether you observe two people expressing love for one another or see a mother embracing her newborn child with loving tenderness, a common theme is witnessed: you observe joy, happiness, and contentment. Opening your heart to love will lead to a life full of joy and happiness.

I remember falling in love when I was thirteen years old. I met this girl from Jackson, Mississippi, who visited my hometown during the summers. I had no idea why I felt the way I did, but I knew that I did not want to be without this girl. I thought about her every second of every day. I could talk to her for hours without getting sleepy or bored. I smiled and blushed when she said my name. Whenever she called, I went running for the phone with joy and enthusiasm. I had no idea what to call these crazy feelings I had, but all I knew is that I hoped that those feelings would never end. Have you ever felt that way about someone before? (Don't act like I was the only one to experience puppy love!)

The truth of the matter is that God wants you to love Him with those same emotions. He wants you to come running joyfully when He calls. He wants you to spend hours talking to Him everyday. He wants you to think about Him every second of every day. God has opened His heart to you. He loves you so much that He continues to give you countless opportunities to improve and to get it right. He wants to delight in your happiness. Take advantage of this opportunity. Open your heart and let His love come inside.

BREAD FOR THE SOUL

Say this prayer and write down any thoughts or requests you have for God:

God, I pray today that You would come into my heart and teach me how to love. I realize that love should be my greatest aim and that without love, I have nothing. Father, I pray that You would instill in me the same love that Jesus has for me. Teach me to love unconditionally and to love the unlovable. Lord, help me to remember all day that life is all about love. Amen.

_____

_____

_____

_____

_____

_____

_____

_____

_____

_____

BREAD FOR THE BODY

Perform thirty minutes of aerobic and anaerobic activity today. Ensure that your workout includes ten minutes of weight and strength training.

Day 3	Exercise Options	What I Did
30 minutes	Free weights	
	Strength training	
	Yoga	
	Aerobics	
	Dumbbells	
	Resistance training	
	Fit for the King DVD	

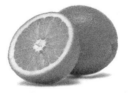

8/6/09

BREAD FOR THE DAY

Day 3	What to Eat	What I Ate
Breakfast	1 cup cereal	
6:30–7:30 a.m.	6 oz. low-fat milk	
	1 hard-boiled egg	
	1 cup cantaloupe	
Mid-morning Snack	¼ cup almonds	
9:30–10:00 a.m.	1 plum	
Lunch	A 4-oz. roast beef sub	
12:00–1:00 p.m.	1 cup coleslaw	
Mid-afternoon Snack	2 celery stalks	
3:00–3:30 p.m.	1 Tbsp. natural peanut butter	
Dinner	A 4-oz. turkey burger	
5:30–8:00 p.m.	1 whole wheat bun	
	1 cup vegetable of choice	
Calories	**1400–1700**	

FAITH

Step 4

BREAD FOR THE MIND

Today's step will require you to take a very long stride. This step is so long that you can actually call it a "leap" of **faith**. We will define *faith* as "confident and unwavering belief in God." How important is having faith in this process?

• **You need faith for success.**

I tell you the truth, if you have faith as small as a mustard seed, you can say to this mountain, "Move from here to there," and it will move. Nothing will be impossible for you. (Matthew 17:20)

• **You need faith for growth.**

Whoever can be trusted with very little can also be trusted with much. (Luke 16:10)

- **You need faith to live right.**

For in the gospel a righteousness from God is revealed, a righteousness that is by faith from first to last, just as it is written: "The righteous will live by faith."   (Romans 1:17)

- **You need faith to please God.**

Without faith it is impossible to please God.
                                        (Hebrews 11:6)

BREAD FOR THE SPIRIT
(Read Hebrews 11:1–12)

One of the hardest things for Christians to do is to believe in the things that our eyes have not yet seen. Most Christians act as though their motto is the same as the State of Missouri's nickname: the "Show Me State." God is not pleased with that attitude! Having total faith in God means that regardless of what you see or believe, you know with complete certainty that God is going to deliver His promises. The Holy Spirit, who lives inside you, is just waiting for you to step out on faith. Make your leap of faith today and watch the change the Holy Spirit makes in you.

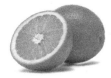

BREAD FOR THE SOUL

Say this prayer and write down any thoughts or requests you have for God:

Father, I know that it is impossible to please You without faith. Help me to learn how to let go and turn everything over to You. I pray that my relationship with You would grow stronger each day, and that through this growth, my faith would grow to enormous proportions. Lord, I love You, and I thank You for Your grace and mercy. Jesus, please use Your Words, Your people, and Your Spirit to help me become more like You. Amen.

_____

_____

_____

_____

_____

_____

_____

_____

_____

_____

_____

_____

BREAD FOR THE BODY

Since we walk by faith and not by sight, I want you to take a thirty- to forty-minute walk. As you walk, take time to reflect on how blessed you are. If you truly think about it, your situation could always be a lot worse. I assure you, there is always someone else with a problem much bigger than yours.

Day 4	Exercise Options	What I Did
30–40 minutes	Walk	
	Jog	
	Power walk	

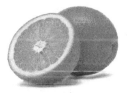

BREAD FOR THE DAY

Day 4	What to Eat	What I Ate
Breakfast	½ cup yogurt w/ granola	
6:30–7:30 a.m.	1 slice toast	
	1 Tbsp. jam or jelly	
	1 peach	
Mid-morning Snack	½ bagel	
9:30–10:00 a.m.	1 tbsp. jam or jelly	
Lunch	A 4-oz. tuna sandwich with lettuce and tomato	
12:00–1:00 p.m.	An 8-oz. garden salad	
Mid-afternoon Snack	2 dill pickles	
3:00–3:30 p.m.		
Dinner	6 oz. grilled salmon	
5:30–8:00 p.m.	1 cup wild rice	
	½ cup carrots	
	½ cup peas	
Calories	**1400–1700**	

HOPE

Step 5

BREAD FOR THE MIND

Does your situation seem hopeless? Then you are probably hanging your hopes on the wrong foundation. Your next step is to put all of your **hope** in the Lord. We will define *hope* as "a confident attitude of expectation." Here's why hope is so important:

- **You need hope for security.**

   You will be secure, because there is hope; you will look about you and take your rest in safety.   (Job 11:18)

- **You need hope for peace of mind.**

   And we know that in all things God works for the good of those who love him, who have been called according to his purpose.   (Romans 8:28)

- **You need hope for strength.**

   Be strong and take heart, all you who hope in the LORD.   (Psalm 31:24)

- **You need hope for your future.**

"For I know the plans I have for you," declares the LORD, "plans to prosper you and not to harm you, plans to give you hope and a future."

(Jeremiah 29:11)

BREAD FOR THE SPIRIT
(Read Romans 8:28–37)

Do you think your situation is hopeless? That may have been the case before you picked up this book. Now that you are on God's path, however, your seemingly hopeless situation just got brighter. If you are alive, you have hope. God is capable of doing anything He has promised. The bottom line is this: as long as you have the ability to look up, you always have hope. What do you hope for? No matter what it is, God can deliver. Keep hope alive!

We know that all things work together for good to those who love God, to those who are the called according to His purpose. (Romans 8:28)

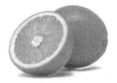

Bread for the Soul

Say this prayer and write down any thoughts or requests you have for God:

Father, help me to place all of my hope in You. I know that with You, all things are possible. No matter what situation I encounter today or what problems I may have, help me to know that everything will be all right. Lord, help me to keep my sights set on heaven so that I will know that there is always hope in You. Amen.

BREAD FOR THE BODY

Perform thirty minutes of aerobic and anaerobic exercise today. Your workout session should target toning your lower body with emphasis on the thighs, hips, and buttocks.

Day 5	Exercise Options	What I Did
30 minutes	Free weights	
	Strength training	
	Aerobics	
	Dumbbells	
	Resistance training	
	Fit for the King DVD	

BREAD FOR THE DAY

Day 5	What to Eat	What I Ate
Breakfast	1 cup oatmeal w/ honey	
6:30–7:30 a.m.	6 oz. low-fat milk	
	2 slices turkey bacon	
	½ cup raisins	
Mid-morning Snack	6 baby carrot sticks	
9:30–10:00 a.m.	1 Tbsp. low-fat ranch dressing	
Lunch	1 peanut butter & jelly sandwich	
12:00–1:00 p.m.	1 banana	
Mid-afternoon Snack	1 granola bar	
3:00–3:30 p.m.	1 peach	
Dinner	4 oz. baked chicken	
5:30–8:00 p.m.	1 baked potato	
	1 Tbsp. sour cream	
	1 cup green beans	
	1 cup squash	
Calories	**1200–1600**	

TRUST

Step 6

BREAD FOR THE MIND

The phrase "In God We Trust" appears on every piece of U.S. currency. That phrase does not mean, "In money we trust," "In family we trust," or "In me I trust." Until now, you have relied on your own abilities to change your situation, to lose weight, or to get in shape. Your next step is to **trust** in God. We will define *trust* as "a confident attitude of reliance." Put your trust in the Lord for:

- **Your Understanding**

  Trust in the LORD with all your heart and lean not on your own understanding.　　　　　(Proverbs 3:5)

- **Your Blessings**

  Blessed is the man who trusts in the LORD, whose confidence is in him.　　　　　(Jeremiah 17:7)

- **Your Happiness**

  May the God of hope fill you with all joy and peace as

*you trust in him, so that you may overflow with hope
by the power of the Holy Spirit.* (Romans 15:13)

- **Your Salvation**

*Surely God is my salvation; I will trust and not be
afraid. The LORD, the LORD, is my strength and my
song; he has become my salvation.* (Isaiah 12:2)

BREAD FOR THE SPIRIT
(Read Psalm 56:1–4)

As Christians, we must understand the intricacies of
Christian trust. You need to trust that the Lord knows what
He is doing, trust that all of your sins have been forgiven,
trust that the Lord will rescue you from all of your troubles,
and trust that He will transform your body into its rightful
shape. Today, I want you to let the lyrics from an old gospel
hymn linger in your minds. The words are very simple:

> *I will trust in the Lord,*
> *I will trust in the Lord,*
> *I will trust in the Lord, until I die.*

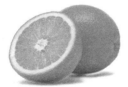

BREAD FOR THE SOUL

Say this prayer and write down any thoughts or requests you have for God:

Lord, help me to trust in You even when my circumstances result in pain. Teach me always to call on You when my situation gets tough. Use my circumstances to mold me to be more like Jesus. Help me to understand that You have a loving purpose in everything that I encounter. Father, help me to trust in You and to understand Your divine purpose for my life. Amen.

_____

_____

_____

_____

_____

_____

_____

_____

_____

_____

_____

_____

BREAD FOR THE BODY

Perform thirty minutes of aerobic and anaerobic activity today. Make sure that your workout includes ten minutes of weight and strength training.

Day 6	Exercise Options	What I Did
30 minutes	Walk	
	Run	
	Treadmill	
	Aerobics	
	Free weights	
	Resistance training	
	Fit for the King DVD	

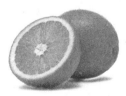

BREAD FOR THE DAY

Day 6	What to eat	What I ate
Breakfast	1 cup cereal	
6:30–7:30 a.m.	6 oz. low-fat milk	
	2 links/patties turkey sausage	
Mid-morning Snack	2 celery stalks	
9:30–10:00 a.m.	1 Tbsp. natural peanut butter	
Lunch	A 4-oz. grilled chicken sandwich on wheat bread	
12:00–1:00 p.m.	1 cup tomato soup	
	1 apple	
Mid-afternoon Snack	¼ cup almonds	
3:00–3:30 p.m.	1 orange	
Dinner	6 oz. grilled scallops	
5:30–8:00 p.m.	1 cup wild rice	
	1 cup mixed veggies	
Calories	**1400–1600**	

SURRENDER

Step 7

BREAD FOR THE MIND

One of the hardest things for people to do is to give up things that they treasure. Today, your seventh step demands that you give up something. Only you know what that thing is. When you **surrender** to Christ, you don't lose; you gain. We will define *surrender* as "the act of relinquishing control to a higher authority." The Lord demands that you surrender:

- **Your Body**

  Therefore, I urge you, brothers, in view of God's mercy, to offer your bodies as living sacrifices, holy and pleasing to God—this is your spiritual act of worship. (Romans 12:1)

- **Your Burdens**

  Cast your cares on the LORD and he will sustain you; he will never let the righteous fall. (Psalm 55:22)

- **Your Devotion to Worldly Possessions**

No one can serve two masters. Either he will hate the one and love the other, or he will be devoted to the one and despise the other. You cannot serve both God and Money. (Matthew 6:24)

- **Your All**

Offer yourselves to God…surrender your whole being to him to be used for righteous purposes.

(Romans 6:13 GNT)

BREAD FOR THE SPIRIT
(Read Romans 6:11–14)

Imagine that you are walking along the street when suddenly a police car stops in front of you. A police officer jumps out, draws his weapon, and points it directly in your face. He yells, "Freeze!" Instinctively, you would probably throw your hands above your head—the universal sign of surrender. Today, the Lord is saying, "Freeze!" You must raise your hands above your head, look to the heavens, and tell God, "I surrender it all to You." Did you do it? Congratulations! Your burdens are about to become much lighter.

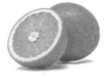

BREAD FOR THE SOUL

Say this prayer and write down any thoughts or requests you have for God:

Lord, I just want to thank You today for pointing me in the right direction. I ask that You would teach me to accept Your help, change my ways, love You deeply, step out in faith, put my hope in Christ, trust in Your plan, and surrender my all to You. Amen.

BREAD FOR THE BODY

When the Lord created the heavens and the earth in six days, He made a point to set aside the seventh day as a day of rest. You must do the same. Today, you should rest your body, relax your mind, and read and reflect on God's Word.

Day 7	Exercises	What I Did
	Rest	
	Read	
	Pray	

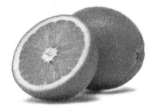

BREAD FOR THE DAY

Day 7	What to Eat	What I Ate
Breakfast	1 cup cereal	
6:30–7:30 a.m.	6 oz. low-fat milk	
	1 hard-boiled egg	
	½ cup raspberries	
Mid-morning Snack	2 large pretzel rods	
9:30–10:00 a.m.	½ cup pineapple	
Lunch	A 4-oz. turkey breast sub on wheat bread with lettuce and tomato	
12:00–1:00 p.m.	1 cup potato salad	
Mid-afternoon Snack	¼ cup almonds	
3:00–3:30 p.m.	1 apple	
Dinner	8 oz. turkey breast	
5:30–8:00 p.m.	1 cup white rice	
	1 cup vegetables	
Calories	**1500–1800**	

Week 2

You Gotta Eat Your Ps!

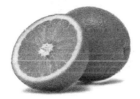

Congratulations! You have successfully completed your first week of Christian weight loss. During your second week, you will have to eat a lot of Ps. Growing up, I would always ask my mother why I had to eat all of my peas. Her response was always the same: "Peas are good for you." Your journey also requires that you consume things that are good for you. I call them the Ps of Christian Nutrition. We will not weigh in at all this week. Your body is going through an adjustment phase, so we are going to let the Lord do His work. I want you to remember that this journey is not about what size *you* think you should be, but what size *God* wants you to be. Remain patient and stay committed!

TESTIMONIALS

"This book is a motivator because it will enhance your confidence and help you to understand the importance of being healthy. I had been struggling with my weight for years. I had tried all types of diet plans with little to no success. Finally, with this plan, I don't feel as though I am dieting—it's more like a spiritual life change; a change that was very much needed. I thank Thomas Hundley for allowing God to lead him in writing this book."

—*Judy Warren*, Harrisburg, North Carolina

"I thoroughly enjoyed the workout DVD. My abdominal area is my trouble spot. I squeezed into a size fourteen when I started; now I'm a comfortable size twelve. I must stress to you: the daily bread for the mind, spirit, soul, and body can become so essential that nothing else matters."

—*Ericka Burrus-Moore,* Columbia, South Carolina

WEEK 2 SHOPPING LIST

List represents meal plan choices and alternatives:

Fresh Vegetables	Fresh Fruits	Canned/ Frozen	Meat	Seafood
17 servings Choose your favorites:	16 servings Choose your favorites:	• Mixed veggies • Minestrone soup • Tomato soup • Vegetable soup • Tuna	• 3 chicken breasts • Ground turkey • Lamb chops • Lunch meat • Turkey bacon	2 servings Choose your favorites:
• Asparagus • Broccoli • Carrots • Cauliflower • Celery • Cucumbers • Green beans • Lettuce • Peppers • Potatoes • Spinach • Sprouts • Squash • Tomatoes • Zucchini Other:	• Apples • Bananas • Blueberries • Cantaloupe • Cherries • Grapes • Kiwis • Melons • Oranges • Peaches • Pears • Plums • Strawberries • Tangerines Other:	Substitutes: • Applesauce • Beans • Beets • Peas • Mixed fruit • Olives • Pickles	Other:	• Crab • Flounder • Halibut • Salmon • Sardines • Scallops • Tilapia • Trout • Tuna steak Other:

Misc. Groceries	Cereal	Dairy	Breads	Snacks
	6 servings Choose your favorites:	• Butter • Eggs • Milk (1% or skim) • Yogurt	• Crackers • English muffins • Whole wheat bread • Wheat wraps	• Almonds • Cashews • Granola bars • Popcorn • Pretzel rods • Raisins • Salsa
• Eggs • Jelly/Jam • Mashed potatoes • Natural peanut butter • Rice • Wild rice • Salad dressings (low-fat) Other:	Cold: • All-Bran • Cheerios • Granola • Grape Nuts • Life • Raisin Bran • Shredded Wheat • Special K Hot: • Cream of wheat • Grits • Oatmeal Other:	Other: • String cheese	Substitutes: • Bagels • Buns • Pita bread • Rolls • Spinach wraps	Substitutes: • Creamsicles • Dried fruit • Multigrain chips • Oatmeal cookies • Protein bars • Special K bars

PRAYER

Step 8

BREAD FOR THE MIND

The first P of Christian nutrition is undoubtedly the most important. This P is your communication link to Christ and your gateway to healing. The only way to the Father is through the Son. The only way to communicate with the Son is through **prayer**. We will define *prayer* as "the act of communicating with God." You must approach prayer in the same manner you approach eating; you must do it several times throughout each day.

- **Pray for blessings.**

  Therefore I tell you, whatever you ask for in prayer, believe that you have received it, and it will be yours.
  (Mark 11:24)

- **Pray for help.**

  I love the LORD, for he heard my voice; he heard my cry for mercy. Because he turned his ear to me, I will call on him as long as I live. (Psalm 116:1–2)

- **Pray for understanding.**

  If any of you lacks wisdom, he should ask God, who gives generously to all without finding fault, and it will be given to him. (James 1:5)

- **Pray for forgiveness.**

  If my people, who are called by my name, will humble themselves and pray and seek my face and turn from their wicked ways, then will I hear from heaven and will forgive their sin and will heal their land.
  (2 Chronicles 7:14)

- **Pray for others.**

  Confess your sins to each other and pray for each other so that you may be healed. The prayer of a righteous man is powerful and effective. (James 5:16)

BREAD FOR THE SPIRIT
(Read Jeremiah 29:11–13)

One of my biggest fears used to be praying aloud or praying before a congregation. I always feared that I would say the wrong things. The fact of the matter was that I wanted to pray like my pastor or deacons, who would just rattle off a resounding prayer as if they were reading it from a book. Then, a good Christian friend taught me the basics of prayer. He had me sit in a chair facing him and told me to close my eyes. Then, he made me tell him everything that was on my mind without opening my eyes. In essence, he was trying to show me that praying to God was no different from having a conversation. You should have a conversation with God every day. When He speaks back and you hear Him, your life will never be the same.

BREAD FOR THE SOUL

Say this prayer and write down any thoughts or requests you have for God:

Father, I thank You for bringing me successfully through my first week of Christian weight loss. Help me to experience and understand the power of prayer. I know that if I open my heart and seek Your righteousness, I will hear Your voice. Speak to me, O Lord, so I may experience Your presence. Amen.

_____

_____

_____

_____

_____

_____

_____

_____

_____

_____

_____

_____

_____

BREAD FOR THE BODY

Perform thirty minutes of cardiorespiratory and/or aerobic activity.

Day 8	Exercise Options	What I Did
30 minutes	Walk	
	Run	
	Treadmill	
	Aerobics	
	Elliptical machine	
	Bicycle	
	Fit for the King DVD	

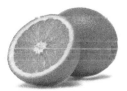

BREAD FOR THE DAY

Day 8	What to Eat	What I Ate
Breakfast	1 cup oatmeal	
6:30–7:30 a.m.	6 oz. low-fat milk	
	2 slices turkey bacon	
	1 peach	
Mid-morning Snack	3 crackers w/natural peanut butter	
9:30–10:00 a.m.	½ cup grapes	
Lunch	A 10-oz. garden salad w/ 2 Tbsp. low-fat dressing	
12:00–1:00 p.m.	1 cup veggie soup	
Mid-afternoon Snack	1 apple	
3:00–3:30 p.m.	½ cup yogurt	
Dinner	4 oz. beef tips	
5:30–8:00 p.m.	½ cup mashed potatoes	
	1 Tbsp. butter	
	1 cup green beans	
Calories	**1500–1800**	

PERSEVERANCE

Step 9

BREAD FOR THE MIND

The second P that you will need is designed to arm you with a weapon to fight off self-doubt. You will face circumstances along your journey that will make you feel like giving up. When you find yourself overwhelmed by a defeatist attitude, you need to grab a bowl of **perseverance**. We will define *perseverance* as "the steadfast continuation of actions in spite of difficulties or setbacks." By taking this weight loss journey, you are doing God's work. Here are the benefits of your steadfast perseverance:

- **Your blessings are within reach.**

  Blessed is the man who perseveres under trial, because when he has stood the test, he will receive the crown of life that God has promised to those who love him. (James 1:12)

- **Your freedom is within reach.**

  Jesus said, "If you hold to my teaching, you are really

my disciples. Then you will know the truth, and the truth will set you free." (John 8:31–32)

- **Your completed mission is within reach.**

The most important thing is that I complete my mission, the work that the Lord Jesus gave me.

(Acts 20:24 NCV)

BREAD FOR THE SPIRIT
(Read 2 Corinthians 4:7–18)

Picture yourself running five miles in order to claim one million dollars. You finally reach the goal and take a step to get your prize when you become distracted by a loud noise. As you pause to see where the noise came from, someone else picks up the money before you can reach it. How would you feel? Don't miss out on your prize because of distractions. You need to push through until the end. Let perseverance be the wind beneath your wings.

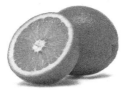

Bread for the Soul

Say this prayer and write down any thoughts or requests you have for God:

Father, although I am sometimes persecuted and suffer despair, I know that You are faithful. I pray that You will provide comfort to me in my times of struggle and in my moments of weakness. Give me the strength and determination to run my race all the way to the end. Amen.

BREAD FOR THE BODY

Perform thirty minutes of aerobic and anaerobic exercise today. Your workout session should target toning your lower body with emphasis on the thighs, hips, and buttocks.

Day 9	Exercise Options	What I Did
30 minutes	Free weights	
	Strength training	
	Aerobics	
	Dumbbells	
	Resistance training	
	Fit for the King DVD	

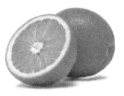

BREAD FOR THE DAY

Day 9	What to eat	What I ate
Breakfast	1 cup cereal	
6:30–7:30 a.m.	6 oz. low-fat milk	
	1 hard-boiled egg	
	½ cup cantaloupe	
Mid-morning Snack	¼ cup almonds	
9:30–10:00 a.m.	1 apple	
Lunch	A 4-oz. grilled chicken wrap	
12:00–1:00 p.m.	6 baby carrots	
	1 Tbsp. low-fat ranch dressing	
Mid-afternoon Snack	3 cups popcorn	
3:00–3:30 p.m.		
Dinner	A 4-oz. turkey burger	
5:30–8:00 p.m.	1 whole wheat bun	
	1 cup vegetable of choice	
Calories	**1400–1700**	

PASSION

Step 10

BREAD FOR THE MIND

Your next serving of Ps will provide fuel for your internal flame. Just like English peas, this P of Christian nutrition is my favorite. Your internal flame may already be a raging fire or it may be a mere flicker. Your internal flame may produce an atomic explosion or it may only produce a controlled detonation. At either rate, your internal flame should be fueled by **passion**. We will define *passion* as "the intense acts of enthusiasm and emotion." The Bible includes wonderful examples of the types of passion you must have.

- **Passion Like David's**

  Zeal for your house consumes me, and the insults of those who insult you fall on me. (Psalm 69:9)

- **Passion Like Paul's**

  I am jealous over you with a jealousy that comes from God. (2 Corinthians 11:2 NCV)

- **Passion Like Christ's**

Whatever you do, work at it with all your heart, as working for the Lord, not for men. (Colossians 3:23)

BREAD FOR THE SPIRIT
(Read Philippians 3:10–15)

Your most important goal should be to please God by developing a closer relationship with Him. God's decree to you, found in Jeremiah 29:13, provides clear-cut guidance: *"You will seek me and find me when you seek me with all your heart."* My simple interpretation of that verse is that if you put all of your heart, passion, and desire into finding God, He will make it worth your effort. You can find God while you try to lose weight. Focus your passions and desires on pleasing God by remaining committed to this plan. I assure you that God will make it worth your effort. Get passionate!

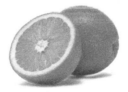

BREAD FOR THE SOUL

Say this prayer and write down any thoughts or requests you have for God:

Dear heavenly Father, give me the passion that I need to seek You with all I have. Help me to develop the desire and determination to stay committed to Your way of life. I strive to live a life that brings glory to You. Amen.

BREAD FOR THE BODY

Perform thirty minutes of aerobic and anaerobic activity today. Make sure that your workout includes ten minutes of weight and strength training.

Day 10	Exercise Options	What I Did
30 minutes	Free weights	
	Strength training	
	Aerobics	
	Dumbbells	
	Resistance training	
	Fit for the King DVD	

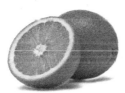

BREAD FOR THE DAY

Day 10	What to Eat	What I Ate
Breakfast	½ cup yogurt w/ granola	
6:30–7:30 a.m.	1 slice wheat toast	
	1 Tbsp. jam or jelly	
	1 banana	
Mid-morning Snack	¼ cup cashews	
9:30–10:00 a.m.	1 plum	
Lunch	A 6-oz. tuna sandwich with lettuce and tomato	
12:00–1:00 p.m.	1 cup minestrone soup	
Mid-afternoon Snack	1 piece string cheese	
3:00–3:30 p.m.	1 pear	
Dinner	6 oz. grilled salmon	
5:30–8:00 p.m.	1 cup wild rice	
	½ cup carrots	
	½ cup asparagus	
Calories	**1400–1800**	

PATIENCE

Step 11

BREAD FOR THE MIND

Right now, you probably need this helping of Ps more than anything else. As Christians, we sometimes become disheartened and lose sight of the ultimate prize. The next step on your journey to weight loss is to develop **patience**. We will define *patience* as "the ability to endure when faced with adversity." This race is not won by the swift but by those who endure to the end. You will need patience to get you to the end of this journey.

- **Patience is a mark of perfection.**

  Let your patience show itself perfectly in what you do. Then you will be perfect and complete and will have everything you need. (James 1:4 NCV)

- **Patience waits for the perfect time.**

  There is a time for everything, and a season for every activity under heaven. (Ecclesiastes 3:1)

- **The Lord has promised to deliver, if we will be patient.**

The message will come true. It may seem like a long time, but be patient and wait for it, because it will surely come; it will not be delayed.

(Habakkuk 2:3 NCV)

BREAD FOR THE SPIRIT
(Read Ecclesiastes 3:1–8)

We live in a world where people want instant results and immediate remedies. It is probably safe to assume that you did not obtain your current size instantly or immediately. Therefore, you must take the same methodical approach to reach the size God wants you to be. When you are tested by the temptations to abandon your journey or cheat on your food choices, remember your P for patience. Those temptations are there only to test you. This is your opportunity to please God by passing the test. If you have doubts or need confirmation, just remember James 1:12: *"Blessed is the man who perseveres under trial, because when he has stood the test, he will receive the crown of life that God has promised to those who love him."* Every day you continue this journey, you will develop more and more Christlike characteristics. Remember, it takes time. And time requires patience.

BREAD FOR THE SOUL

Say this prayer and write down any thoughts or requests you have for God:

Dear Lord, help me to remember that the temptations that I face are only tests of my will. Teach me to approach each circumstance and every temptation with patience and understanding. Help me to respond in a manner that pleases You and brings glory to Your kingdom. Amen.

BREAD FOR THE BODY

It's time to walk it out! Today, go for a long walk. If you are able, mix in a light jog with the walking. The objective for today is to get out and get moving for at least thirty minutes. Use this time to reflect on the areas in your life where more patience on your part is required.

Day 11	Exercise Options	What I Did
30–40 minutes	Walk	
	Jog	
	Power walk	

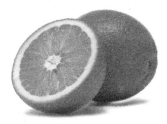

BREAD FOR THE DAY

Day 11	What to Eat	What I Ate
Breakfast	1 cup cereal	
6:30–7:30 a.m.	6 oz. low-fat milk	
	½ cup raspberries	
Mid-morning Snack	1 granola bar	
9:30–10:00 a.m.	1 banana	
Lunch	A 4-oz. turkey sandwich on wheat bread	
12:00–1:00 p.m.	1 cup vegetable soup	
Mid-afternoon Snack	2 large pretzel rods	
3:00–3:30 p.m.	6 strawberries	
Dinner	6 oz. baked fish	
5:30–8:00 p.m.	1 cup broccoli	
	1 baked potato	
	2 Tbsp. salsa	
Calories	**1500–1800**	

Step 12

BREAD FOR THE MIND

At this stage on your journey, you need a little comfort food. You may feel overwhelmed or discouraged at various points along this journey. You may be overcome by a series of emotions that cause you discomfort. The next P that you must develop is **peace**. We will define *peace* as "a state of spiritual calm and serenity." This journey requires that you develop peace for:

- **Your Heart**

  Let the peace of Christ rule in your hearts, since as members of one body you were called to peace. And be thankful.　　　　　　　　　　(Colossians 3:15)

- **Your Strength**

  The LORD gives strength to his people; the LORD blesses his people with peace.　　　　　　　　　(Psalm 29:11)

- **Your Service**

  Whatever you have learned or received or heard from

me, or seen in me—put it into practice. And the God of peace will be with you. (Philippians 4:9)

- **Your Comfort**

Peace I leave with you; my peace I give you. I do not give to you as the world gives. Do not let your hearts be troubled and do not be afraid. (John 14:27)

BREAD FOR THE SPIRIT
(Read Isaiah 26:1–4)

While serving in the military in Iraq, I once found myself caught in the midst of a firestorm of mortars. Like an Olympic sprinter, I ran for the nearest cement bunker. As I reached it, I found that I was alone. Panic, fear, and anxiety quickly set in as the mortars continued to explode all around me. Immediately, I bowed my head and prayed to God to help me remain calm during this time. In an instant, twelve young soldiers made their way to the bunker. It was easy to see that they were more afraid and confused than I was. Being the highest ranking soldier in the bunker, I was thrust into a role of responsibility. I instinctively took charge of the group by laying out a plan of how we would proceed. As I spoke to them, my fear and anxiety disappeared. When the attack ended, I realized that the Lord had actually answered my prayer. I had prayed for Him to help me remain calm and He gave me an opportunity to exhibit calmness. Trust the Lord to give you peace during your storms.

BREAD FOR THE SOUL

Say this prayer and write down any thoughts or requests you have for God:

Father, when the storms of life are raging, I pray that You will provide my heart with a sense of peace and calm. Teach me to trust in Your grace and mercy to see me through the most challenging of situations. More than anything else, Lord, help me to serve as a source of peace for others. I know that Your love and peace will endure forever. Amen.

BREAD FOR THE BODY

Perform thirty minutes of aerobic and anaerobic exercise today. Your workout session should target toning your lower body with emphasis on the thighs, hips, and buttocks.

Day 12	Exercise Options	What I Did
30 minutes	Free weights	
	Strength training	
	Aerobics	
	Dumbbells	
	Resistance training	
	Fit for the King DVD	

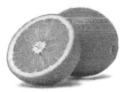

BREAD FOR THE DAY

Day 12	What to Eat	What I Ate
Breakfast	1 cup oatmeal w/ raisins	
6:30–7:30 a.m.	6 oz. low-fat milk	
	2 slices turkey bacon	
Mid-morning Snack	6 baby carrot sticks	
9:30–10:00 a.m.	1 Tbsp. ranch dressing	
Lunch	1 natural peanut butter & jelly sandwich	
12:00–1:00 p.m.	1 banana	
Mid-afternoon Snack	1 granola bar	
3:00–3:30 p.m.	1 peach	
Dinner	6 oz. baked chicken	
5:30–8:00 p.m.	1 cup white rice	
	½ cup green beans	
	½ cup squash	
Calories	**1200–1600**	

PRAISE

Step 13

BREAD FOR THE MIND

It is now time to for you to consume a P that satisfies your appetite. The Lord is making slow and steady changes in your life. The things that you have accomplished, and those you are about to accomplish, are not of your own doing. For that reason, you have to remember to consume an abundance of the next P on your weight-loss journey. You must remember to always give God the **praise**. We will define *praise* as "the act of expressing admiration and appreciation for God's great works." Here is how to praise the Lord:

- **Praise Him with your heart.**

  I will praise you, O LORD, with all my heart; I will tell of all your wonders. (Psalm 9:1)

- **Praise Him with your mouth.**

  I will be glad and rejoice in You; I will sing praise to Your name, O Most High. (Psalm 9:2)

- **Praise Him with your soul.**

I praise you because I am fearfully and wonderfully made; your works are wonderful, I know that full well. (Psalm 139:14)

BREAD FOR THE SPIRIT
(Read Psalm 126)

O Praise Him! O Praise Him! For He is worthy to be praised! Growing up, I remember people often beginning their testimonies by saying, "First, I give honor to God, who is the head of my life." I often wondered why people said that and what it really meant. It was not until I experienced God's greatness that I truly understood what those people were saying. Now I begin every day with that same sentiment. It is my way of praising God and thanking Him for being the guiding force in my life. I realize that He is the reason for every move I make and every breath I take. As you go through your day, make sure that you take time to give God His proper praise. He is most definitely worthy of your praise and more.

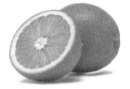

BREAD FOR THE SOUL

Say this prayer and write down any thoughts or requests you have for God:

Father, how I sing Your praises for Your magnificent works! I fully understand that I could not accomplish anything in my life without You. I realize that You are the source of my being and the source of my strength. Thank You for bringing me this far along in my journey. I know that You will see me through until the end. Amen.

BREAD FOR THE BODY

Perform thirty minutes of cardiorespiratory and/or aerobic activity.

Day 13	Exercise Options	What I Did
30 minutes	Walk	
	Run	
	Treadmill	
	Aerobics	
	Elliptical machine	
	Bicycle	
	Fit for the King DVD	

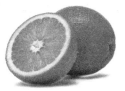

BREAD FOR THE DAY

Day 13	What to Eat	What I Ate
Breakfast	1 cup cereal	
6:30–7:30 a.m.	6 oz. low-fat milk	
	½ cup raspberries	
Mid-morning Snack	2 celery stalks	
9:30–10:00 a.m.	1 Tbsp. natural peanut butter	
Lunch	1 turkey & ham sandwich on wheat bread	
12:00–1:00 p.m.	½ cup tomato soup	
Mid-afternoon Snack	¼ cup almonds	
3:00–3:30 p.m.	1 orange	
Dinner	6 oz. baked lamb chop	
5:30–8:00 p.m.	½ cup wild rice	
	1 cup mixed vegetables	
Calories	**1400–1600**	

PURPOSE

Step 14

BREAD FOR THE MIND

I remember the day that I finally put together all of the pieces of the puzzle of life. Everything started to make sense as I answered those really bizarre questions I often asked myself. *Why am I short? Why do I look younger than my age? Why do complete strangers find it easy to discuss their personal problems with me?* I must admit, that last question baffled me for years. I often wondered if my chosen profession should have been that of a psychiatrist.

This next step is so important that the Lord is directing me to take a different approach. I am going to share my personal testimony of how I found my purpose. Your final P along this journey represents the dessert of your meal—to find and understand your **purpose**. We will define *purpose* as "the reason for your existence." Instead of giving you several points to ponder, I am going to share the story of how I found my own purpose for existing.

BREAD FOR THE SPIRIT
(Read Ephesians 1:3–12)

There is no better feeling in the world than knowing and understanding God's purpose for your life. In December 2004, I took my own forty-day spiritual journey by reading *The Purpose Driven Life* by Rick Warren. I discovered that my purpose on earth was to be a servant leader. Going through that journey caused me to begin seeking direction by reading the Bible. It was within those pages that I began hearing God's voice, understanding His words, and applying His instructions.

Over the course of the next two years, the Lord placed me in positions of increased responsibility. These new positions helped me to grow closer to Him and helped to prepare me for this very moment. On April 29, 2004, while attending the 9:30 a.m. service at Friendship Missionary Baptist Church in Charlotte, North Carolina, the Lord spoke to me. His voice was undeniable and unmistakable. As I prayed to God, He said, "I have chosen you for a mission. You will share My Good News while helping the church to improve its heath and physical fitness. You are well prepared." I opened my eyes and looked around to see if anyone else in church had heard what I heard. I smiled to myself, and I verbally replied to God, "Yes, Lord, send me and I'll go."

To confirm that this actually happened and was not a mere figment of my mind, as we prepared for the benediction, the pastor, Dr. Clifford A. Jones Sr., stated, "I cannot leave without saying this to you all. The Holy Spirit is telling me that someone in here just got their calling from the Lord. He is telling me that the Lord just gave someone in here a mission. My advice to you is that you had better listen and obey, because you may never get another opportunity like this." With those words ringing in my head, I went home and began writing down everything the Lord wanted me to do. The first task He gave me was to record a workout video that combined Christianity with fitness. You are currently reading the results of the second task the Lord commissioned me to do.

To better understand why you are reading this book, you need to know about some of the events that led to this point. In February 2004, I began to neglect church fellowship by using Sundays to spend more time with my family. I could sense that the Lord was calling me, but I was purposely ignoring His call. A month later, my boss informed me that I had to move to Fort Bragg, North Carolina, within the coming months to participate in Operation Iraqi Freedom. My family and I had been in San Antonio, Texas, for only fifteen months, and it was very strange that we were being asked to leave so soon. My wife and I decided that the best thing to do was for me to leave them in San Antonio and to go to Fort Bragg by myself. I believe this was the Lord's way of separating me from my family so He could begin His work in me without distractions. You see, the Lord does not want you to have anyone or anything before Him, including your family. (See Matthew 10:37–38).

While in Iraq, I begin to develop an even closer relationship with God. I began teaching a *Purpose Driven Life* Bible study twice a week—I had only been to one Bible study in my life. My classes grew in attendance from eight people to forty people. The Lord was preparing me by forcing me to learn His Word so that I could better instruct others. I began singing with the praise and worship team—and I can't even sing!

More than ever, I was carrying myself as a child of God. I wanted every part of my life to be more like Christ.

For the next three hundred twenty-seven days that I served in Iraq, my life revolved around three main priorities: serving God, serving my country, and getting physically fit. As I developed my body into a lean, mean, fighting machine, others began to take notice. Two soldiers asked me to help them with their workouts. I found myself again thrust into a teaching and mentoring role. I was forced to learn as much as possible about physical fitness to better instruct my group on proper training. To my surprise, not only were our workouts extremely effective for weight loss, but they were also motivating, entertaining, and inspiring. Eventually, I was able to help more than forty soldiers and airmen reach their fitness goals by following these workouts.

In November 2005, I returned home from Iraq a changed man. My family moved from San Antonio to Charlotte, North Carolina, which was much closer to my base. With my newfound passion for physical fitness, I began to teach aerobics classes. I found great enjoyment in helping others lose weight while having a good time doing it. After a full year of perfecting my technique, my style of training, and my skills, the Lord spoke those words to me that set me in motion: "You are well prepared."

I know the purpose that the Lord has for my life through this ministry. I have no doubt that this fitness ministry will be extremely successful in bringing people closer to Christ. I have no doubt that this ministry will also help people find their God-given sizes and shapes. God speaks to me daily, providing me with specific instructions on how to lead this ministry. There are times when doubt and uncertainty creep into my mind. I initially wondered where I would get the money to finance this project. But every time there was a cost or expense, the Lord provided the exact amount needed. Now, my fears and doubt have turned into courage and confidence. The Lord has stated repeatedly through His Word, *"Never will I leave you; never will I forsake you"* (Hebrews 13:5; see also Deuteronomy 31:6, 8; Joshua 1:5). Philippians 4:19 states, *"My God will meet all your needs according to his glorious riches in Christ Jesus."* All I have to do now is respond obediently to what I hear and be resilient in what I do.

The Lord has blessed me with the secret to healthy Christian living and physical fitness. He has prepared and sent me to share it with you. The joy you will experience at the end of this journey will completely change your life. You will find that your life is more satisfying, more enjoyable, and so much easier. I encourage you to get a copy of *The Purpose Driven Life* by Rick Warren. It is no coincidence that the number forty appears so many times in this book, in Rick Warren's book, and also in the Bible. It is a number that represents a journey or trial. It was the number of years Israel wandered in the desert. It was the number of days Jesus spent being tempted in the wilderness. It was also the number of days the risen Lord spent on earth after the resurrection. You are experiencing internal and external changes right now as you read these pages. The Lord has placed you where He needs you to be. It's time for you to find your purpose.

BREAD FOR THE SOUL

Say this prayer and write down any thoughts or requests you have for God:

> Lord, I was made by You and I know that You know what's best for me. Help me to discover my purpose in You. Jesus, I want to learn to think like You, walk like You, speak like You, and act the way You would act. Help me, Lord, to focus my mind and my life on what You have called me to do. Amen.

BREAD FOR THE BODY

Today is your day to rest and reflect. Think about those things that make you different from everyone else in the world. You should think deeply and intently about the things you have experienced throughout your life. Make a list of questions concerning your body and your life that you never understood. This is your day to work mentally on your life's puzzle.

Day 14	Exercise Options	What I Did
	Rest	
	Read	
	Pray	

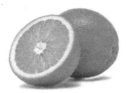

BREAD FOR THE DAY

Day 14	What to Eat	What I Ate
Breakfast	1 cup cereal	
6:30–7:30 a.m.	6 oz. low-fat milk	
	2 slices turkey bacon	
	1 banana	
Mid-morning Snack	1 cup grapes	
9:30–10:00 a.m.		
Lunch	An 8-oz. salad	
12:00–1:00 p.m.	2 Tbsp. low fat Caesar dressing	
	1 cup veggie soup	
Mid-afternoon Snack	½ English muffin	
3:00–3:30 p.m.	1 tsp. jam or jelly	
Dinner	6 oz. grilled chicken	
5:30–8:00 p.m.	1 cup wild rice	
	1 cup green beans	
Calories	**1400–1700**	

Week 3

YOU GOTTA BUILD SOME CHRISTIAN MUSCLE!

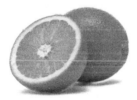

Congratulations! You have successfully completed your second week of Christian weight loss. If you have been faithful in your commitment to this journey, I am certain that you have noticed some physical changes in your body. This is only the beginning. During the coming week, we will increase the intensity of our spiritual and physical training. You will find yourself doing things that will develop and build your Christian muscle.

Before beginning your readings for today, take a moment to weigh yourself. Record your weight and today's date below. Stay encouraged, because this is just the beginning!

Date: _____

Weight: _____

TESTIMONIALS

"I am sixty years old with high blood pressure and type 2 diabetes. Not only is this a good diet, but it's also helping me to eat right. When I started this diet, I weighed two hundred seventy-one pounds. After week two, I weighed two hundred sixty-one pounds. At the end of my forty-day journey, I weighed an even two hundred fifty pounds. More importantly, I lost three dress sizes. God has a special anointing on this book and on Thomas Hundley."

—*Shirley Palmer*, Columbia, South Carolina

"I have been a big girl all of my life. I have tried every plan under the sun, but I could never stick to anything. This book has helped me to understand that God made me to be a big girl, but He demands that I be healthy. I lost twenty-two pounds after week five, but more importantly, I know that my size is supposed to be a fourteen. I can live with that!"

—*Donnie Johnson*, Tacoma, Washington

WEEK 3 SHOPPING LIST

List represents meal plan choices and alternatives:

Fresh Vegetables	Fresh Fruits	Canned/Frozen	Meat	Seafood
16 servings Choose your favorites:	14 servings Choose your favorites:	• Peas • Pickles • Soups • Tomatoes • Tuna • Vegetable soup	• 3 chicken breasts • Cube steak • Ground turkey • Lunch meat • Turkey bacon • Turkey breast	1 serving Choose your favorite:
• Asparagus • Beets • Broccoli • Carrots • Cauliflower • Celery • Cucumbers • Green beans • Lettuce • Peppers • Potatoes • Spinach • Squash • Tomatoes • Zucchini Other:	• Apples • Bananas • Blueberries • Cantaloupe • Cherries • Grapes • Kiwis • Melons • Oranges • Peaches • Pears • Plums • Raspberries • Strawberries • Tangerines Other:	Substitutes: • Applesauce • Beans • Beets • Carrots • Mixed fruit • Mixed veggies • Olives	Other:	• Crab • Flounder • Halibut • Salmon • Sardines • Scallops • Tilapia • Trout • Tuna steak Other:

Misc. Groceries	Cereal	Dairy	Breads	Snacks
• Coleslaw • Jelly/Jam • Natural peanut butter • Potato salad • Salad dressings (low-fat) • White rice • Wild rice Other:	6 servings Choose your favorites: Cold: • All-Bran • Cheerios • Grape Nuts • Life • Raisin Bran • Shredded Wheat • Special K Hot: • Cream of wheat • Grits • Oatmeal Other:	• Eggs • Margarine • Milk (1% or Skim) • Yogurt Other:	• Buns • Crackers • English muffins • Whole wheat bread • Rolls Substitutes: • Bagels • Pita bread • Spinach wraps • Wheat wraps	• Almonds • Cashews • Granola bars • Popcorn • Pretzel rods • Salsa Substitutes: • Creamsicles • Dried fruit • Multigrain chips • Oatmeal cookies • Protein bars • Raisins • Special K bars

STRENGTH

Step 15

BREAD FOR THE MIND

The Lord created you with a predetermined purpose in mind. God planned your life to be used for a very important mission. To complete that mission, you will need a certain amount of **strength** along the way. We will define *strength* as "the spiritual, physical, and emotional toughness required to deal with situations." The next step on your Christian weight loss journey requires you to develop strength of various kinds:

- **Spiritual Strength**

  I pray that out of his glorious riches he may strengthen you with power through his Spirit in your inner being. (Ephesians 3:16)

- **Physical Strength**

  He gives strength to the weary and increases the power of the weak....Those who hope in the LORD will renew their strength. They will soar on wings like eagles; they will run and not grow weary, they will walk and not be faint. (Isaiah 40:29, 31)

- **Prayer Strength**

The Spirit helps us in our weakness. We do not know what we ought to pray for, but the Spirit himself intercedes for us with groans that words cannot express.

(Romans 8:26)

- **Strength in Christ**

I can do everything through him who gives me strength. (Philippians 4:13)

BREAD FOR THE SPIRIT
(Read Psalm 46:1–7)

You possess something greater than strength. You have the power of the almighty God who made the heavens and the earth. You have the power of prayer that can move mountains. You have the strength of Christ, who said that His grace is sufficient for you. I wish I could eloquently articulate how strong you are with God on your side. When you experience a moment of weakness, take a moment to say a simple prayer that will get you through. Simply say, "Lord, give me strength." Repeat it as much as you need to. Jesus has promised that anything you ask for in His name He will do. (See John 14:13.) It really does not matter where you are in life, in your relationships, in your career, or in this weight loss journey. The Lord will meet you right where you are and give you the strength to go on.

BREAD FOR THE SOUL

Say this prayer and write down any thoughts or requests you have for God:

Father, give me strength during the times when I am weak. Give me strength when my burdens feel too heavy to carry. Give me the strength to carry on when my situations and circumstances seem hopeless. I know that with faith, I can do all things through Christ who gives me strength. Amen.

BREAD FOR THE BODY

Perform thirty minutes of aerobic and anaerobic activity today. Ensure that your workout includes ten minutes of weight and strength training.

Day 15	Exercise Options	What I Did
30 minutes	Free weights	
	Strength training	
	Aerobics	
	Dumbbells	
	Resistance training	
	Fit for the King DVD	

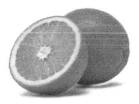

BREAD FOR THE DAY

Day 15	What to Eat	What I Ate
Breakfast	1 cup cereal	
6:30–7:30 a.m.	6 oz. low-fat milk	
	2 slices turkey bacon	
	1 apple	
Mid-morning Snack	6 crackers w/ natural peanut butter	
9:30–10:00 a.m.		
Lunch	A 10-oz. salad w/ 2 Tbsp. low-fat Caesar dressing	
12:00–1:00 p.m.	1 cup veggie soup	
Mid-afternoon Snack	¼ cup cashews	
3:00–3:30 p.m.	1 banana	
Dinner	6 oz. grilled chicken	
5:30–8:00 p.m.	1 cup wild rice	
	1 cup green beans	
	1 dinner roll	
Calories	**1400–1700**	

ENDURANCE

Step 16:

BREAD FOR THE MIND

You have come too far to give up now. This is the time to take that deep breath and press forward. As a Christian, you will encounter pitfalls and booby traps along your way. When you face these obstacles, don't give up. You have to keep running the race to the end. With that said, your next step is to develop some Christian **endurance**. We will define *endurance* as "the ability to tolerate prolonged challenges." Here's why you must develop endurance.

- **Your freedom awaits.**

  Therefore, since we are surrounded by such a great cloud of witnesses, let us throw off everything that hinders and the sin that so easily entangles, and let us run with perseverance the race marked out for us.

  (Hebrews 12:1)

- **Your purpose awaits.**

  Not that I have already attained, or am already perfected; but I press on, that I may lay hold of that for which Christ Jesus has also laid hold of me.

  (Philippians 3:12 NKJV)

- **Your crown awaits.**

Blessed is the man who perseveres under trial, because when he has stood the test, he will receive the crown of life that God has promised to those who love him. (James 1:12)

BREAD FOR THE SPIRIT
(Read Philippians 3:13–21)

You know, and have probably heard, that the race is not won by the swift, but by he who endures to the end. On your journey, the same saying applies. You are blessed beyond measure right now. The Lord is waiting for you to prove your commitment, obedience, and faithfulness. When you take one step, He will take two. No matter how tough your road may seem today, tomorrow, or this week, you must weather the storm. Your ability to endure during trying times will please God immensely. And when you please God with your actions, He will definitely please you with His. Hang in there and keep looking up.

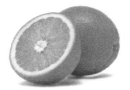

BREAD FOR THE SOUL

Say this prayer and write down any thoughts or requests you have for God:

Dear heavenly Father, I come to You, thanking You for keeping me on the right path thus far. I pray that You will see me through until the end of my journey. There is so much that awaits me at the end of this race. Please help me to keep my focus on the eternal and not on the temporary. Amen.

BREAD FOR THE BODY

Perform thirty minutes of cardiorespiratory and/or aerobic activity.

Day 16	Exercise Options	What I Did
30 minutes	Walk	
	Run	
	Treadmill	
	Aerobics	
	Elliptical machine	
	Bicycle	
	Fit for the King DVD	

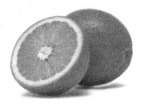

BREAD FOR THE DAY

Day 16	What to Eat	What I Ate
Breakfast	1 cup cereal	
6:30–7:30 a.m.	6 oz. low-fat milk	
	½ cup raspberries	
	1 hard-boiled egg	
Mid-morning Snack	2 large pretzel rods	
9:30–10:00 a.m.	½ cup pineapple	
Lunch	A 4-oz. turkey breast sub on wheat bread	
12:00–1:00 p.m.	1 cup potato salad	
Mid-afternoon Snack	¼ cup almonds	
3:00–3:30 p.m.	1 apple	
Dinner	6 oz. grilled scallops	
5:30–8:00 p.m.	½ cup white rice	
	1 cup asparagus	
	1 dinner roll	
Calories	**1500–1700**	

DESIRE

Step 17

BREAD FOR THE MIND

What do you have an intense longing for? What do you want more than anything else? The answers to those questions are vital to your next step. The Lord repeatedly tells you in His Word that He wants you to seek Him with all of your heart. He commands you to love Him above all others, to love Him with all your heart, with all your soul, and with all your mind. (See Matthew 22:37.) When you do this, you have successfully taken the step of **desire**. We will define *desire* as "an extreme longing or aspiration for something or someone." Your goal right now is to find, focus, and fulfill your deepest desires.

- **Find the desire to love God.**

  Love the LORD your God with all your heart and with all your soul and with all your strength.

  (Deuteronomy 6:5)

- **Focus on the desires of your heart.**

  For where your treasure is, there your heart will be also. (Matthew 6:21)

120

- **Fulfill your desire to finish your journey.**

*We desire that each one of you show the same dili-
gence to the full assurance of hope until the end, that
you do not become sluggish, but imitate those who
through faith and patience inherit the promises.*

(Hebrews 6:11–12 NKJV)

- **Receive your reward.**

Delight yourself in the LORD *and he will give you the
desires of your heart.* (Psalm 37:4)

BREAD FOR THE SPIRIT
(Read Romans 8:1–8)

God can change your life in amazing ways when you put
Him first. I am sitting here writing a book because I know
this is what God wants. My greatest desire is to please Him
with my life. I offer myself to Him to be used in whatever
capacity He chooses. He has chosen to use me to reach others through health and fitness instruction. He is going to use
me to help others come to know Him by showing His power
through weight loss. I have found my desire to please God,
focused my heart on fitness and nutrition, and fulfilled my
desire to finish my mission. Today, I bask in the glow of having received my reward. Now it is your turn. You must find,
focus, and fulfill the desires of your heart.

BREAD FOR THE SOUL

Say this prayer and write down any thoughts or requests you have for God:

Lord, it is my deepest desire to please You. If there is anything that I am placing before You, please help me to see the error of my ways. Please help me to focus less on worldly desires and more on heavenly desires. Father, I ask You to help me to find those true desires within my heart so that You can use me to serve Your purpose. Amen.

_____

_____

_____

_____

_____

_____

_____

_____

_____

_____

_____

_____

_____

BREAD FOR THE BODY

Perform thirty minutes of aerobic and anaerobic exercise today. Your workout session should target toning your lower body with emphasis on the thighs, hips, and buttocks.

Day 17	Exercise Options	What I Did
30 minutes	Free weights	
	Strength training	
	Aerobics	
	Dumbbells	
	Resistance training	
	Fit for the King DVD	

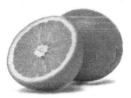

BREAD FOR THE DAY

Day 17	What to Eat	What I Ate
Breakfast	1 cup cereal	
6:30–7:30 a.m.	6 oz. low-fat milk	
	½ cup raspberries	
	1 hard-boiled egg	
Mid-morning Snack	2 cups popcorn	
9:30–10:00 a.m.	1 plum	
Lunch	A 4-oz. turkey breast sub on wheat bread	
12:00–1:00 p.m.	1 Tbsp. low-fat dressing	
	4 celery stalks	
Mid-afternoon Snack	¼ cup almonds	
3:00–3:30 p.m.	1 apple	
Dinner	6 oz. turkey breast	
5:30–8:00 p.m.	½ cup white rice	
	1 cup spinach	
	1 cup squash	
Calories	**1600–1800**	

COURAGE

Step 18

BREAD FOR THE MIND

When confronted with a challenge, do you back down or rise up? If you find yourself backing down more often than standing up, then it is time for you to take a very important step in your Christian life. No matter how overwhelming your situation may be, you have the ultimate backup in Jesus. He will provide you with the **courage** to face your situation and win. We will define *courage* as "the ability to overcome fear." Jesus has already fought your battle for you. So, go forth and be courageous!

- **You've got protection.**

  But, Lord, you are my shield, my wonderful God who gives me courage. (Psalm 3:3 NCV)

- **You've got companionship.**

  Be strong and courageous, and do the work. Do not be afraid or discouraged, for the LORD God, my God, is with you. (1 Chronicles 28:20)

- **You've got support.**

  Do not fear, for I am with you; do not be dismayed, for I am your God. I will strengthen you and help you.
  (Isaiah 41:10)

- **You've got Christ.**

  Yes, my dear children, live in him so that when Christ comes back, we can be without fear and not be ashamed in his presence. (1 John 2:28 NCV)

BREAD FOR THE SPIRIT
(Read Hebrews 12:1–13)

Nike's slogan, "Just Do It!" is exactly what God has been telling His chosen people for centuries. When Moses had to cross the Red Sea, God said, "Just do it!" When Noah had to build the ark, God said, "Just do it!" When David faced Goliath, God said, "Just do it!" When Daniel was thrown in the lions' den, God said, "Just do it!" Those examples serve as the blueprints of courage that you need to build on right now. Don't think for a second that Daniel, Moses, and David were any different from you. You, too, have been chosen by God to do an equally important mission. When you are fully prepared, the Lord is going to reveal your mission and your purpose. To accomplish that mission, you will need a strong dose of courage. But don't fear! The Lord has told you in His Word that no weapon formed against you shall prevail. (See Isaiah 54:17.) So, why worry or have doubts about this Christian weight loss journey? The Lord is telling you, "Just do it!"

BREAD FOR THE SOUL

Say this prayer and write down any thoughts or requests you have for God:

Lord, give me the courage to break out of my comfort zone so You can use me to fulfill Your purpose. Help me to know and understand that You are with me even in my darkest times. When I am confronted with life's challenges, help me to rise to the occasion and live victoriously. Father, give me the courage to "Just Do It!" Amen.

BREAD FOR THE BODY

Perform thirty minutes of aerobic and anaerobic exercise today. Your workout session should target toning your lower body with emphasis on the thighs, hips, and buttocks.

Day 18	Exercise Options	What I Did
30 minutes	Free weights	
	Strength training	
	Aerobics	
	Dumbbells	
	Resistance training	
	Fit for the King DVD	

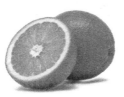

BREAD FOR THE DAY

Day 18	What to Eat	What I Ate
Breakfast	1 cup cereal	
6:30–7:30 a.m.	6 oz. low-fat milk	
	½ cup raisins	
Mid-morning Snack	1 granola bar	
9:30–10:00 a.m.	1 banana	
Lunch	A 4-oz. turkey sandwich on wheat bread	
12:00–1:00 p.m.	An 8-oz. garden salad	
	2 Tbsp. low-fat dressing	
Mid-afternoon Snack	1 cup strawberries	
3:00–3:30 p.m.		
Dinner	6 oz. baked fish	
5:30–8:00 p.m.	1 cup broccoli	
	1 baked potato	
	1 cup beets	
Calories	**1500–1800**	

CONFIDENCE

Step 19

BREAD FOR THE MIND

Now that you have found your courage and strength in the Lord, it is time to show the world your glow. By this point in your journey, you are probably feeling a little lighter externally and a lot cleaner internally. This should produce a radiant glow in your complexion. Believe me, someone is going to notice. Your next step is to further develop your **confidence**. We will define *confidence* as "belief in your own abilities." Walk with your head high and your shoulders back. You are a child of the King, which means you are an heir of royalty. Be majestic today. The Holy Spirit is in you and God is smiling on you. Your step for today is to be confident! This confidence is rooted in these truths:

- **You are protected.**

  I will instruct you and teach you in the way you should go; I will counsel you and watch over you.

  (Psalm 32:8)

- **You are purposeful.**

  And we know that in all things God works for the

130

good of those who love him, who have been called according to his purpose. (Romans 8:28)

- **You are powerful.**

*You, dear children, are from God and have overcome them, because the one who is in you **is greater** than the one who is in the world.*

(1 John 4:4, emphasis added)

BREAD FOR THE SPIRIT
(1 Corinthians 4:1–4)

I remember a scene from the movie *The Nutty Professor* with Eddie Murphy that has a profound impact on the way I counsel clients. The protagonist, Buddy Love, was having a conversation on the subject of confidence with Ms. Carla Purty, played by Jada Pinkett-Smith. In the scene, Buddy said, "I tell Sherman all the time that he needs to suck in his gut and strut." Now, although Eddie Murphy's comments may seem a little insensitive, I think they carry an important message for Christian living. As Christians, we are living representatives of the almighty God. It is our obligation, therefore, to walk with our chests out as we perform God's work. It is our duty to speak boldly as we deliver the Good News. It is your responsibility to *"present yourself to God as one approved, a workman who does not need to be ashamed"* (2 Timothy 2:15). You have been well equipped and well prepared, so be the confident person God has made you to be.

BREAD FOR THE SOUL

Say this prayer and write down any thoughts or requests you have for God:

Dear Lord, I know that I am a child of God, and that fact alone makes me special. Create in me the confidence I need to step out in faith and do the impossible. Lord, I ask that You would place one person in my path today who notices the spirit You have made alive in me. I pray that You would use me to make a difference in someone's life today. Amen.

BREAD FOR THE BODY:

Perform thirty minutes of cardiorespiratory and/or aerobic activity.

Day 19	Exercise Options	What I Did
30 minutes	Walk	
	Run	
	Treadmill	
	Aerobics	
	Elliptical machine	
	Bicycle	
	Fit for the King DVD	

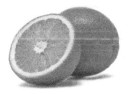

BREAD FOR THE DAY

Day 19	What to Eat	What I Ate
Breakfast	1 slice wheat toast	
6:30–7:30 a.m.	½ cup yogurt with fruit	
	1 Tbsp. jam or jelly	
Mid-morning Snack	¼ cup almonds	
9:30–10:00 a.m.	1 plum	
Lunch	A tuna sandwich on wheat bread	
12:00–1:00 p.m.	1 cup coleslaw	
	1 Tbsp. low-fat dressing	
Mid-afternoon Snack	2 cups popcorn	
3:00–3:30 p.m.	1 pear	
Dinner	6 oz. cubed steak	
5:30–8:00 p.m.	1 cup wild rice	
	½ cup carrots	
	½ cup peas	
Calories	**1400–1700**	

RESTRAINT

Step 20

BREAD FOR THE MIND

Confidence helps to develop character. Each day, the Lord is helping you to develop Christlike character by the fruit of the Spirit. (See Galatians 5:22–23.) So far, the Lord has given you love, peace, faithfulness, and patience. As you continue on your journey, you will also receive joy and kindness. Having these types of fruit in your life will help you to become more like Christ. But merely having these characteristics is not enough. You will not simply wake up tomorrow morning and instantly display love or patience. The Lord has to develop the fruit by giving you opportunities to grow. He will place you in situations where you will display either the fruit of the Spirit or the exact opposite characteristics.

The one question you should ask yourself in all situations is, *What would Jesus do?* You've probably heard this phrase and even seen the acronym on bracelets, various articles of clothing, and even bumper stickers. Nevertheless, the question is valid: *What **would** Jesus do?*

Your next step is to develop **restraint**. We will define *restraint* as "the act of displaying self-control." When you face temptations in life (notice I said *when*, and not *if*), remember to ask yourself, *What would Jesus do?*

- **God produces a test; you produce the temptation.**

  When tempted, no one should say, "God is tempting me." For God cannot be tempted by evil, nor does he tempt anyone; but each one is tempted when, by his own evil desire, he is dragged away and enticed.
  (James 1:13–14)

- **God provides options; you make the decisions.**

  No temptation has seized you except what is common to man. And God is faithful; He will not let you be tempted beyond what you can bear. But when you are tempted, he will also provide a way out so that you can stand up under it. (1 Corinthians 10:13)

- **God rewards success; you pass the test.**

  Blessed is the man who perseveres under trial, because when he has stood the test, he will receive the crown of life that God has promised to those who love him. (James 1:12)

- **God showed you "the way"; you follow "the life."**

  For we do not have a high priest who is unable to sympathize with our weaknesses, but we have one [Jesus] who has been tempted in every way, just as we are—yet was without sin. (Hebrews 4:15)

BREAD FOR THE SPIRIT
(Read Galatians 5:16–26)

"Run, Forrest, run!" We all have heard that line from the movie *Forrest Gump*. In the movie, when Forrest faced trouble or danger, his friends would often tell him just to run away as fast as he could. As your brother in Christ, I am giving you the same advice. Defeating temptations in life is no easy task. The temptations I speak of are not the singing group who crooned, "Ain't Too Proud to Beg." Rather, our temptations come in the forms of sexual immorality, lust, hatred, jealousy, drunkenness, envy, selfish ambitions, and *food*. This list is not all-inclusive. Only you know the specific temptations that you battle in life.

The Lord will give you plenty of opportunities to defeat your temptations. He has given you the ability to choose. The best way to defeat a temptation is by making the right choice. With every victory—or right choice—you grow a step closer to Christ.

I have my own formula for defeating temptations. Because I love you and want to see you succeed, I am going to share it with you. I use the "5-R Method." For example, if I enter a room where I am immediately tempted, here is how it works:

- **Recognize:** I recognize when I am in a vulnerable situation. *"Uh-oh! This may not be the best place for me to be right now."*

- **Request:** I request God's help immediately. *"Lord, I think I'm going to need Your help to get out of this one. I need some strength right now."*

- **Remember:** I remember the letters WWJD. *"Okay Thomas, think! What would Jesus do? What would Jesus do?"*

- **Recite:** I recite a verse to refocus my attention on something other than my temptation. *"The LORD is my shepherd...." "For it is written...."*

- **Run:** I run away from that situation as fast as I can. *"Run, Thomas, run! I'm outta here. Peace!"*

Remember, God gives you the gift of choice. When you make the right choice, He smiles and rewards you for your decisions. When you make the wrong choice, He gives you another opportunity to make the right choice. That is the beauty of God's grace and mercy. He loves you so much that He forgives you and gives you another opportunity to grow. Build your resistance and practice restraint today.

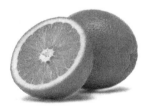

BREAD FOR THE SOUL

Say this prayer and write down any thoughts or requests you have for God:

Father God, thank You for loving me so much that You give me opportunities to grow. Thank You for entrusting me with Your precious gift of choice. Help me to recognize and resist temptation so that I can become more like Christ. Help me to respond to temptations in the same manner that Jesus would. Father, continue to develop the fruit of the Spirit in my life. Amen.

BREAD FOR THE BODY

Perform thirty minutes of aerobic and anaerobic activity today. Ensure that your workout includes ten minutes of weight and strength training.

Day 20	Exercise Options	What I Did
30 minutes	Free weights	
	Strength training	
	Aerobics	
	Dumbbells	
	Resistance training	
	Fit for the King DVD	

BREAD FOR THE DAY

Day 20	What to Eat	What I Ate
Breakfast	1 cup cereal	
6:30–7:30 a.m.	6 oz. low-fat milk	
	½ cup raisins	
	1 hard-boiled egg	
Mid-morning Snack	¼ cup almonds	
9:30–10:00 a.m.	1 apple	
Lunch	A 4-oz. grilled chicken sub w/ low-fat dressing	
12:00–1:00 p.m.	1 cup potato salad	
Mid-afternoon Snack	2 celery stalks	
3:00–3:30 p.m.	1 Tbsp. natural peanut butter	
Dinner	A 6-oz. turkey burger	
5:30–8:00 p.m.	½ cup white rice	
	½ cup carrots	
	1 whole wheat bun	
Calories	**1500–1800**	

COMMITMENT

Step 21

BREAD FOR THE MIND

Your Christian muscle development is almost complete. Now, you need to build the one Christian muscle that ties all the others together. This muscle should be stronger than all of the others because it strengthens all of the others. The next step on your Christian weight loss journey is to develop your **commitment** to Christ. We will define *commitment* as "the unwavering dedication to serving God." When you possess a strong commitment to serving God, He will strengthen your desire, boost your confidence, build your courage, and develop your self-control. You will then have the endurance you need to complete this journey. Be committed to Christ!

- **Commitment = Support**

  Commit your way to the LORD; trust in him and he will do this: He will make your righteousness shine like the dawn, the justice of your cause like the noon-day sun.   (Psalm 37:5–6)

- **Commitment = Success**

  Commit to the LORD whatever you do, and your plans will succeed.   (Proverbs 16:3)

- **Commitment = Self-worth**

Do your best to present yourself to God as one approved, a workman who does not need to be ashamed and who correctly handles the word of truth.

(2 Timothy 2:15)

- **Commitment = Salvation**

He gave himself for us so he might pay the price to free us from all evil and to make us pure people who belong only to him—people who are always wanting to do good deeds. (Titus 2:14 NCV)

BREAD FOR THE SPIRIT
(Read Romans 12:1–8)

At the beginning of this book, I asked you to sign a contract—your forty-day commitment to completing this journey. The Lord wants you to sign a similar contract with Him. Each day, He assigns you small tasks to test your faithfulness, as well as your commitment to larger ones. Many people make casual promises and commitments only to break them at the slightest inconvenience or trouble. I have always wondered why over 50 percent of marriages end in divorce. Think about it. You stand in church (the body of Christ) and make a vow to stay with that person until you die, regardless of finances, health, or other circumstances. Real commitment means you weather the storm and fulfill your promise. God is giving you an opportunity to show your faithfulness and commitment today. When you pass this forty-day test, He has something greater waiting for you at the end. He is just waiting to say to you,

Well done, good and faithful servant! You have been faithful with a few things; I will put you in charge of many things. Come and share your master's happiness!
(Matthew 25:23)

BREAD FOR THE SOUL

Say this prayer and write down any thoughts or requests you have for God:

Father, help me to live a life of service to You by holding true to my promises. Help me to care faithfully for the small things You place in my life so that I can learn how to handle the larger ones. Lord, thank You for shaping me to serve You. Today I recommit my life to being like Christ. Amen.

_____

_____

_____

_____

_____

_____

_____

_____

_____

_____

_____

BREAD FOR THE BODY

Today is your rest day! You should think about how powerful you are going to be now that you have Christian muscle. Read and reflect on God's Word!

Day 21	Exercise Options	What I Did
	Rest	
	Read	
	Pray	

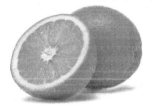

BREAD FOR THE DAY

Day 21	What to Eat	What I Ate
Breakfast	1 cup oatmeal	
6:30–7:30 a.m.	6 oz. low-fat milk	
	2 slices turkey bacon	
	1 apple	
Mid-morning Snack	6 crackers w/natural peanut butter	
9:30–10:00 a.m.		
Lunch	An 8-oz. salad	
12:00–1:00 p.m.	2 Tbsp. low-fat Caesar dressing	
	1 cup vegetable soup	
Mid-afternoon Snack	¼ cup cashews	
3:00–3:30 p.m.	1 banana	
Dinner	6 oz. grilled chicken	
5:30–8:00 p.m.	1 baked potato w/ 2 Tbsp. salsa	
	1 cup green beans	
	1 dinner roll	
Calories	**1500–1700**	

Week 4

YOU GOTTA GET SOME SOUL FOOD!

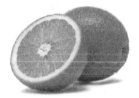

Congratulations! You have successfully completed your third week of Christian weight loss. By now, you are probably experiencing a difference in the way your clothes fit. You may also begin to notice some positive, physical changes in your body. If so, take a moment to celebrate by giving God the praise.

Okay, now that you have celebrated, let's get back to work. You have nineteen more days to go, and I don't want you to grow complacent with your accomplishments. There is an even bigger miracle waiting for you at the end of this journey. Over the course of the next week, you will incorporate some of God's "Soul Food" into your diet.

Once again, we will skip the weigh-in for today. Whatever you do, please resist the urge to get on the scale. Just relish in the fact that your clothes are fitting better. Stay humble and stay committed!

TESTIMONIALS

"I just finished my third week. And, I cheated today! I weighed myself. It was one of those *I'm in a doctor's office, so why not* kind of things. To my amazement, I have lost thirteen pounds. What a boost! This is the first time something like this has worked, and it doesn't involve spending three hours in a gym, running until I'm wheezing, starving myself, or eating cottage cheese and cabbage soup. What a godsend."

—*Andrea Brazil*, Eastover, South Carolina

"I love the way this book is designed, especially the inspirational thoughts along with Scripture, which help to put things into perspective. I have lost fifteen pounds after twenty-one days and my clothes are way too loose. This plan is so simple to follow that I can hardly wait to read the next day's message. I can't wait for the next book."

—*John Loper*, Waynesboro, Mississippi

WEEK 4 SHOPPING LIST
List represents meal plan choices and alternatives:

Fresh Vegetables	Fresh Fruits	Canned/ Frozen	Meat	Seafood
18 servings Choose your favorites:	18 servings Choose your favorites:	• Peas • Mixed veggies • Pickles • Tuna	• 4 chicken breasts • Lamb chops • Lunch meat • Turkey bacon • Turkey breast	2 servings Choose your favorites::
• Asparagus • Broccoli • Carrots • Cauliflower • Celery • Cucumbers • Green beans • Lettuce • Peppers • Potatoes • Spinach • Sprouts • Squash • Tomatoes • Zucchini (Other:	• Apples • Bananas • Blueberries • Cantaloupe • Cherries • Grapes • Kiwis • Melons • Oranges • Peaches • Pears • Plums • Raspberries • Strawberries • Tangerines Other:	Substitutes: • Applesauce • Beans • Beets • Carrots • Mixed fruit • Olives • Soups • Tomatoes	Other:	• Crab • Flounder • Halibut • Salmon • Sardines • Scallops • Tilapia • Trout • Tuna steak Other:

Misc. Groceries	Cereal	Dairy	Breads	Snacks
• Baked potato chips • Jelly/Jam • Natural peanut butter • White rice • Wild rice • Salad dressings (low-fat) Other:	6 servings Choose your favorites: Cold: • All-Bran • Cheerios • Grape Nuts • Life • Raisin Bran • Shredded Wheat • Special K Hot: • Cream of wheat • Grits • Kasha • Oatmeal Other:	• Eggs • Milk (1% or skim) • Sour cream • Yogurt Other:	• Bagels • Crackers • English muffins • Whole wheat bread • Pita bread • Rolls • Spinach wraps Substitutes: • Buns • Rolls • Wheat wraps	• Almonds • Granola bars • Oatmeal cookies • Wheat pretzels Substitutes: • Cashews • Creamsicles • Dried fruit • Multigrain chips • Popcorn • Protein bars • Raisins • Salsa • Special K bars

GRACE

Step 22

BREAD FOR THE MIND

For the next week, you will be experiencing the wonderful gifts of God that are used to feed your soul—hence the name "Soul Food." The Lord provides His "soul food" to you in abundance and at no cost or obligation. Essentially, following your Christian weight loss journey is taking a trip through God's free buffet line. The first item you need to put on your plate is **grace**. We will define *grace* as "God's gift of unearned forgiveness." Here are the nutritional benefits of God's grace:

- **God's grace is loving.**

  But God, who is rich in mercy, because of His great love with which He loved us, even when we were dead in trespasses, made us alive together with Christ (by grace you have been saved).

  (Ephesians 2:4–5 NKJV)

- **God's grace is patient.**

Being confident of this very thing, that He who has begun a good work in you will complete it until the day of Jesus Christ. (Philippians 1:6 NKJV)

- **God's grace is powerful.**

My grace is sufficient for you, for my power is made perfect in weakness. (2 Corinthians 12:9)

- **God's grace is compassionate.**

Now I commit you to God and to the word of his grace, which can build you up and give you an inheritance among all those who are sanctified. (Acts 20:32)

BREAD FOR THE SPIRIT
(Romans 5:1–8)

God freely gives His grace to us even though we don't deserve it. You can go through your entire life doing good deeds for others, preaching the gospel seven days a week, and feeding the homeless in your spare time, and still you would be undeserving of God's grace. Indeed, the beauty of God's grace is that you don't have to earn it—you couldn't if you tried. You are only required to repent (see Step 2), have faith (see Step 4), and pray (see Step 8). As of now, you are a recipient of God's grace. Please do not take this gift of God lightly—it is precious and sacred. Be thankful, grateful, and faithful. Congratulations! You have just taken a giant step on the road to sanctification (becoming more like Christ), as well as a giant leap on the path of righteousness.

BREAD FOR THE SOUL

Say this prayer and write down any thoughts or requests you have for God:

Dear heavenly Father, I thank You for giving me Your precious gift of grace. I am so thankful that You love me despite my shortcomings. Help me, Lord, to do all I can with what You have given me. I pray that the Holy Spirit would continually help me to remember to treat Your gift of grace as a sacred trust. Amen.

BREAD FOR THE BODY:

Perform thirty minutes of cardiorespiratory and/or aerobic activity. I recommend taking a speed walk.

Day 22	Exercise Options	What I Did
30 minutes	Walk	
	Run	
	Treadmill	
	Aerobics	
	Elliptical machine	
	Bicycle	
	Fit for the King DVD	

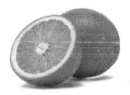

BREAD FOR THE DAY

Day 22	What to Eat	What I Ate
Breakfast	1 cup oatmeal	
6:30–7:30 a.m.	6 oz. low-fat milk	
	2 slices turkey bacon	
	1 apple	
Mid-morning Snack	6 crackers w/ jam	
9:30–10:00 a.m.	1 pear	
Lunch	A 10-oz. garden salad w/ 2 Tbsp. low-fat dressing	
12:00–1:00 p.m.	1 cup vegetable soup	
Mid-afternoon Snack	½ English muffin	
3:00–3:30 p.m.	1 Tbsp. jelly	
Dinner	6 oz. grilled chicken	
5:30–8:00 p.m.	1 cup wild rice	
	1 cup green beans	
Calories	**1500–1800**	

MERCY

Step 23

BREAD FOR THE MIND

Now that you have the main course of God's soul food meal on your plate, you need to choose some side items. Just as turkey goes well with stuffing, steak with potatoes, and chicken with rice, grace is best served with a side of God's **mercy**. We will define *mercy* as "God's gift of undeserved compassion." God displays this gift in many ways:

- **In Times of Trouble**

  I will be glad and rejoice in your mercy, for You have considered my trouble; You have known my soul in adversities. (Psalm 31:7 NKJV)

- **In Times of Faithfulness**

  I thank Christ Jesus our Lord, who has given me strength, that he considered me faithful, appointing me to his service. Even though I was once a blasphemer

155

and a persecutor and a violent man, I was shown mercy because I acted in ignorance and unbelief.
(1 Timothy 1:12–13)

· In Times When You Show Mercy

Religion that God our Father accepts as pure and faultless is this: to look after orphans and widows in their distress and to keep oneself from being polluted by the world. (James 1:27)

· In Times of His Choosing

For [God] says to Moses, "I will have mercy on whom I have mercy, and I will have compassion on whom I have compassion." It does not, therefore, depend on man's desire or effort, but on God's mercy.
(Romans 9:15–16)

BREAD FOR THE SPIRIT
(Read Matthew 27–31)

The Bible gives many examples of ways that God demonstrated His mercy. He used His Son, Jesus, to heal blind men and lepers and to awaken those who were pronounced dead. As we are not worthy of God's grace, we likewise are not worthy of God's mercy. Yet God is compassionate and freely shows us mercy when we break His commandments or disobey His Word.

I believe that God's mercy is best shown in ways in which we are not even aware. When I was a teenager, I recall being upset because my mother established an 11:00 p.m. curfew. All my friends were allowed to hang out until at least midnight. Naturally, I felt that I was being denied the freedom that my friends frequently enjoyed. I remember voicing my frustrations with my great-grandmother, who quickly dropped some of her sage wisdom on me. "Son," she said, "you should be thankful because it's not always what God gets you out of, but more so what He keeps you from getting into." I have since learned that she was so right. Be thankful that you serve a merciful God.

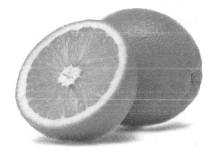

BREAD FOR THE SOUL

Say this prayer and write down any thoughts or requests you have for God:

Father, how great is Your mercy toward me that it always abides in me! How great is Your mercy for me and how great is Your grace! Lord, I thank You for all of the trials You brought me through and all of the trials You've kept me from. Help me to use the mistakes and failures in my life to better understand Your mercy. Amen.

BREAD FOR THE BODY

Perform thirty minutes of aerobic and anaerobic exercise today. Your workout session should target toning your lower body with emphasis on the thighs, hips, and buttocks.

Day 23	Exercise Options	What I Did
30 minutes	Free weights	
	Strength training	
	Aerobics	
	Dumbbells	
	Resistance training	
	Fit for the King DVD	

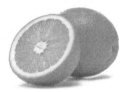

BREAD FOR THE DAY

Day 23	What to Eat	What I Ate
Breakfast	1 cup cereal	
6:30–7:30 a.m.	6 oz. low-fat milk	
	1 oz. raisins	
	1 slice toast w/ 1 Tbsp. jam	
Mid-morning Snack	1 granola bar	
9:30–10:00 a.m.	1 banana	
Lunch	A 4-oz. turkey sandwich w/ lettuce and tomato	
12:00–1:00 p.m.	1 oz. baked potato chips	
Mid-afternoon Snack	4 wheat pretzels	
3:00–3:30 p.m.	6 strawberries	
Dinner	4 oz. baked fish	
5:30–8:00 p.m.	1 cup broccoli	
	1 baked potato	
	1 Tbsp. sour cream	
Calories	**1500–1800**	

FORGIVENESS

Step 24

BREAD FOR THE MIND

You have just piled your plate with grace and mercy. A good soul food meal, however, needs even more side dishes. The next step on your journey requires that you stack your plate with God's **forgiveness**. We will define *forgiveness* as "God's gift of excusing our sins." God's greatest gift to us was His Son, Jesus, who died that our sins would be forgiven. The Bible provides your proof:

- **Jesus bled for your forgiveness.**

   In Him we have redemption through His blood, the forgiveness of sins, according to the riches of His grace. (Ephesians 1:7 NKJV)

- **Jesus died for your forgiveness.**

   And he died for all, that those who live should no longer live for themselves but for him who died for them and was raised again. (2 Corinthians 5:15)

- **Jesus was resurrected for your forgiveness.**

  It shall be imputed to us who believe in Him who raised up Jesus our Lord from the dead, who was delivered up because of our offenses, and was raised because of our justification. (Romans 4:24–25 NKJV)

- **Jesus forgets the reasons you need forgiveness.**

  For I will forgive their wickedness and will remember their sins no more. (Hebrews 8:12)

BREAD FOR THE SPIRIT
(Read Matthew 18:21–35)

One of the most generous and gracious gifts the Lord provides is the gift of forgiveness. He created you in His own image and entrusted you to care for His creation. Your past decisions may not have demonstrated good stewardship, but all is not lost. Right now, God is showing you His grace, His mercy, and His forgiveness through this book. You are being afforded another opportunity to show God that you can be trusted. No matter how great your mistakes, your shortcoming, or your sin, God forgives you. *Yes*, He forgives you for that thing nobody else knows about. *Yes*, He forgives you for that thing you think you got away with. *Yes*, He even forgives you for those things you only *thought* about doing. Now, it's time for you to forgive yourself.

While I was in Iraq, I met a young lady who seemed to be deep in thought. Something about her just begged for me to engage her in conversation. Being that I have never been short on casual conversation, I talked to her. Less than five minutes into our conversation, the young lady revealed that she had committed a sin for which she could not forgive herself. She said that her husband knew all about her sin and was deeply hurt by her actions. To her surprise, she stated that her husband was willing to forgive her and wanted to work things out. She could not understand how one whom she had hurt so deeply could forgive her and still love her despite her shortcomings. Her major problem was that she had not forgiven herself. Her husband was a man of God. His willingness and ability to forgive and love his wife demonstrated his Christlike character.

This is exactly what God does for us every day of our lives. As we approach the cross in repentance, He sees our sin, sheds a tear, forgives our sin, and loves us all the more.

Think about this—you can relieve yourself of your burdens today by just asking for forgiveness. God's love for you is unconditional. All He wants is for you to tell Him that you did wrong, tell Him what you did wrong, and then ask Him for forgiveness. Once God forgives you, He forgets that it ever happened—*and so should you!*

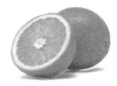

BREAD FOR THE SOUL

Say this prayer and write down any thoughts or requests you have for God:

Lord, I pray for Your forgiveness today. Help me to let go of those thoughts and memories that continue to keep me from being like Christ. Help me to find it in my heart to forgive myself for the wrongs I've done and to forgive those who have done wrong to me. I thank You for Your precious gift of forgiveness. Amen.

BREAD FOR THE BODY

Perform thirty minutes of aerobic and anaerobic activity today. Ensure that your workout includes ten minutes of weight and strength training.

Day 24	Exercise Options	What I Did
30 minutes	Free weights	
	Strength training	
	Aerobics	
	Dumbbells	
	Resistance training	
	Fit for the King DVD	

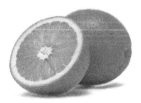

BREAD FOR THE DAY

Day 24	What to Eat	What I Ate
Breakfast	1 cup cereal	
6:30–7:30 a.m.	6 oz. low-fat milk	
	1 hard-boiled egg	
	1 cup cantaloupe	
Mid-morning Snack	¼ cup almonds	
9:30–10:00 a.m.	1 apple	
Lunch	1 grilled chicken wrap	
12:00–1:00 p.m.	2 Tbsp. low-fat ranch dressing	
	6 baby carrots	
Mid-afternoon Snack	2 celery sticks	
3:00–3:30 p.m.	1 Tbsp. natural peanut butter	
Dinner	6-oz. turkey burger	
5:30–8:00 p.m.	½ cup white rice	
	1 cup spinach	
	1 whole wheat bun	
Calories	**1500–1800**	

DELIVERANCE

Step 25

BREAD FOR THE MIND:

Your soul food plate is filling up, but it is not quite full. After receiving God's grace, mercy, and a double helping of forgiveness, you will need a serving of redemption. The next step on your weight loss journey is to get God's **deliverance**. We will define *deliverance* as "God's gift of redemption and rescue." This gift of God gives you freedom, and the price for your freedom was paid in full.

- **Delivered from Trouble**

  Then they cried out to the LORD in their trouble, and he delivered them from their distress. (Psalm 107:6)

- **Delivered from Shame**

  For I know that through your prayers and the help given by the Spirit of Jesus Christ, what has happened to me will turn out for my deliverance. I eagerly expect and hope that I will in no way be ashamed, but will have sufficient courage so that now as always Christ will be exalted in my body, whether by life or by death. (Philippians 1:19–20)

- ### Delivered from Sin

But thanks be to God that, though you used to be slaves to sin, you wholeheartedly obeyed the form of teaching to which you were entrusted. You have been set free from sin and have become slaves to righteousness. (Romans 6:17–18)

- ### Delivered for Good

If the Son sets you free, you will be free indeed. (John 8:36)

BREAD FOR THE SPIRIT
(Read Psalm 107:1–9)

You have just received God's gift of deliverance. To help you understand fully what that means, I must paint a picture for you. Imagine yourself holding a big box in your hands. Inside this box is a flat-screen TV that weighs seventy-five pounds. Your task is to carry that box up seven flights of stairs. You march up the stairs one by one. By the time you reach the fifteenth step, you're feeling the weight of the box. The higher you go, the heavier the box seems to get. You reach step twenty and your arms begin to shake. You reach step twenty-five and someone takes the box from you, offering to carry it the rest of the way. Can you feel the weight on your arms being released? Can you imagine taking a big breath and releasing a sigh of relief? Today, on the twenty-fifth step of your Christian weight loss journey, the Lord has just freed you from your shackles, rescued you from your situations, and delivered you from your sin. You should shout to the world, "I'm free at last, free at last, thank God almighty, I'm free at last."

BREAD FOR THE SOUL

Say this prayer and write down any thoughts or requests you have for God:

Lord, thank You for Your gift of freedom. I thank You for the freedom from guilt, the freedom from our past sins, and the freedom from our burdens. Teach me to stand strong and to continue to keep my eyes on the prize. Father, continue to remind me of how far I've come, not how far I still have to go. I thank You for helping me to remain committed to my journey. Amen.

_____

_____

_____

_____

_____

_____

_____

_____

_____

_____

BREAD FOR THE BODY:

Perform thirty minutes of aerobic and anaerobic exercise today. Your workout session should target toning your lower body with emphasis on the thighs, hips, and buttocks.

Day 25	Exercise Options	What I Did
30 minutes	Free weights	
	Strength training	
	Aerobics	
	Dumbbells	
	Resistance training	
	Fit for the King DVD	

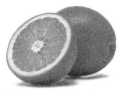

BREAD FOR THE DAY

Day 25	What to Eat	What I Ate
Breakfast	1 slice toast w/ 1 Tbsp. jam	
6:30–7:30 a.m.	½ cup yogurt w/ granola	
	1 orange	
Mid-morning Snack	½ bagel w/ jam	
9:30–10:00 a.m.	1 plum	
Lunch	A 4-Oz. tuna sandwich	
12:00–1:00 p.m.	1 Tbsp. low-fat dressing	
	2 celery stalks	
Mid-afternoon Snack	1 granola bar	
3:00–3:30 p.m.	1 pear	
Dinner	6 oz. grilled salmon	
5:30–8:00 p.m.	½ cup wild rice	
	½ cup carrots	
	½ cup green peas	
Calories	**1400–1700**	

JOY

Step 26

BREAD FOR THE MIND

It is a known fact that soul food provides comfort and happiness. I can't think of many things that bring me happiness like that of banana pudding and sweet potato pie. Your next step requires that you get some of God's comfort food in the form of **joy**. We will define *joy* as "God's gift of gladness and delight." You may experience many things in life that bring you temporary happiness, but you obtain *eternal* happiness when you experience God's gift of joy.

- **Morning Joy**

  Weeping may endure for a night, but joy comes in the morning.　　　　　(Psalm 30:5 NKJV)

- **Rewarding Joy**

  Well done, good and faithful servant! You have been faithful with a few things; I will put you in charge of many things. Come and share your master's happiness!　　　　　(Matthew 25:21)

- **Situational Joy**

Sorrowful, yet always rejoicing; poor, yet making many rich; having nothing, and yet possessing every-thing. (2 Corinthians 6:10)

- **Unspeakable Joy**

But the fruit of the Spirit is love, joy, peace, patience, kindness, goodness, faithfulness, gentleness and self-control. Against such things there is no law.
(Galatians 5:22–23)

BREAD FOR THE SPIRIT
(Read Psalm 30:4–12)

It is very important for you understand what it means to have joy in your life. Don't confuse *joy* with *happiness*. There is a distinct difference between these two emotions. In the Bible, the word *happiness* is found six times. The word *joy* is found two hundred forty-two times (forty times more—again, there's that number). The Lord was so serious about wanting you to know the meaning of joy that He said it twice through the apostle Paul: *"Rejoice in the Lord always. I will say it again: Rejoice!"* (Philippians 4:4).

I want to tell you about the two most significant friends ever to enter my life: Happiness and Joy. Happiness was the friend who came into my life, put a smile on my face, and made my days brighter. Happiness was a great friend to have around, but when I needed Happiness most, Happiness always seemed to be too busy. You see, Happiness had a serious aversion to commitment and an allergic reaction to trouble. So, my Happiness was here today and gone tomorrow.

My friend, Joy, came into my life and not only put a smile on face, but also put a smile on my heart. With Joy, not only were my days brighter, but my life was also brighter. I could always count on Joy being there for me. When Happiness was in my life, Joy was there, too. When Happiness left, Joy was still there. I guess it was no surprise when Joy said to me, "Thomas, I will be with you for better or for worse, in sickness and in health, until death do us part." It dawned on me that Joy was the permanent cure for my temporary Happiness. I am proud to say that I have been living a life full of Joy ever since.

The Lord wants you to live a joyful life. Just ask Him for it and watch Him deliver. Remember, being happy does not necessarily mean that you are joyful, but being joyful means you have eternal happiness.

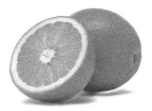

BREAD FOR THE SOUL

Say this prayer and write down any thoughts or requests you have for God:

Lord, I am asking You right now to bring joy into my life. Bless me with a heart of contentment and a lifetime of happiness. Fill me with the joy that can be found only by knowing Your Son, Jesus. Help me to realize that happiness is only temporary, but Your exceeding joy is eternal. Father, teach me to rejoice in the Lord always; again, I say, "Rejoice!" Amen.

BREAD FOR THE BODY

Perform thirty minutes of aerobic and anaerobic activity today. Ensure that your workout includes ten minutes of weight and strength training.

Day 26	Exercise Options	What I Did
30 minutes	Free weights	
	Strength training	
	Aerobics	
	Dumbbells	
	Resistance training	
	Fit for the King DVD	

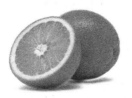

BREAD FOR THE DAY

Day 26	What to Eat	What I Ate
Breakfast	1 cup oatmeal	
6:30–7:30 a.m.	6 oz. low-fat milk	
	2 slices turkey bacon	
	½ grapefruit	
Mid-morning Snack	6 baby carrots	
9:30–10:00 a.m.	1 Tbsp. low-fat ranch dressing	
Lunch	1 natural peanut butter & jelly sandwich	
12:00–1:00 p.m.	1 orange	
Mid-afternoon Snack	1 granola bar	
3:00–3:30 p.m.	1 peach	
Dinner	4 oz. baked chicken	
5:30–8:00 p.m.	1 baked potato	
	1 cup green beans	
	1 Tbsp. sour cream	
Calories	**1500–1700**	

SALVATION

Step 27

BREAD FOR THE MIND

No soul food meal would ever be complete without a little dessert. The sweetest gift that the Lord offers you is the gift of **salvation.** We will define *salvation* as "God's gift of deliverance from sin." The Lord gave us all the greatest gift of all in His Son, Jesus Christ. Through Jesus, we are offered an opportunity to experience redemption for our sins. Your next weight loss step requires you to receive the gift of salvation. If you've already received salvation from God through Christ, it never hurts to go through the process again and to thank God for what He has done in your life. Here's how to receive the gift of salvation:

- **Realize that you are a sinner.**

  For all have sinned and fall short of the glory of God, and are justified freely by his grace through the redemption that came by Christ Jesus.

  (Romans 3:23–24)

- **Read the Bible for direction.**

From childhood you have known the Holy Scriptures, which are able to make you wise for salvation through faith which is in Christ Jesus. (2 Timothy 3:15 NKJV)

- **Exhibit faith in God.**

It is by grace you have been saved, through faith— and this not from yourselves, it is the gift of God.
(Ephesians 2:8)

- **Confess and believe in Jesus.**

If you confess with your mouth, "Jesus is Lord," and believe in your heart that God raised him from the dead, you will be saved. For it is with your heart that you believe and are justified, and it is with your mouth that you confess and are saved.
(Romans 10:9–10)

BREAD FOR THE SPIRIT
(Read Colossians 1:12–18)

Today is an important and dramatic step in your life. By accepting God's gift of salvation, you become an heir to a life of abundance. You are making the choice to accept health over sickness, peace over chaos, love over hate, and life over death. By accepting salvation—by confessing that Jesus is your personal Savior—you gain permanent control over your weight problem. Now, your problems become Jesus' problems. Jesus is asking for an opportunity to help you to solve this problem. Today, turn all of your weight loss and health burdens over to Jesus. All it takes is saying—and meaning— these words:

Lord, I believe in Your Son, Jesus Christ. I believe that Jesus died for my sins and that You raised Him from the dead. Lord, I accept Jesus as my personal Savior.

Congratulations! You have just won the most important battle in the war of life.

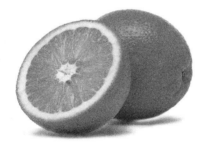

BREAD FOR THE SOUL

Say this prayer and write down any thoughts or requests you have for God:

God, I come to You in the name of Jesus, asking for forgiveness of my sins. From this day forward, I desire to establish a close and personal relationship with Jesus. Come into my heart and cleanse me of my guilt and embarrassment for the sins I have committed. I pray that You would make me into the person You intended me to be. I humbly receive Christ as my Savior and my Lord. Amen.

_____

_____

_____

_____

_____

_____

_____

_____

_____

_____

_____

BREAD FOR THE BODY:

Perform thirty minutes of cardiorespiratory and/or aerobic activity.

Day 27	Exercise Options	What I Did
30 minutes	Walk	
	Run	
	Treadmill	
	Aerobics	
	Elliptical machine	
	Bicycle	
	Fit for the King DVD	

BREAD FOR THE DAY

Day 27	What to Eat	What I Ate
Breakfast	1 cup cereal	
6:30–7:30 a.m.	6 oz. low-fat milk	
	1 hard-boiled egg	
	1 oz. raisins	
Mid-morning Snack	2 celery stalks	
9:30–10:00 a.m.	1 Tbsp. natural peanut butter	
Lunch	A 4-oz. turkey sandwich on whole wheat bread	
12:00–1:00 p.m.	½ cup tomato soup	
	1 apple	
Mid-afternoon Snack	½ cup almonds	
3:00–3:30 p.m.	1 orange	
Dinner	A 4-oz. lamb chop	
5:30–8:00 p.m.	1 cup wild rice	
	1 cup carrots	
	1 oatmeal cookie	
Calories	**1500–1700**	

VICTORY

Step 28

BREAD FOR THE MIND

Only one thing remains to make your soul food experience complete. You have consumed God's entire meal for your soul, but you still need something to wash it down. The next step on your journey is to consume a bottle of a refreshing, invigorating beverage called **victory**. We will define *victory* as "God's gift of personal celebration." You have cause to celebrate. The Lord has taken your problems; He is fighting your battles; He is giving you a new body. All you have to do is the following:

- **Believe in Him.**

Everyone born of God overcomes the world. This is the victory that has overcome the world, even our faith. Who is it that overcomes the world? Only he who believes that Jesus is the Son of God.

(1 John 5:4–5)

- **Have faith in Him.**

And we know that in all things God works for the

good of those who love him, who have bee called according to his purpose. (Romans 8:28)

- **Thank Him.**

Thanks be to God! He gives us the victory through our Lord Jesus Christ. (1 Corinthians 15:57)

- **Praise Him.**

Oh, sing to the LORD a new song! For He has done marvelous things; His right hand and His holy arm have gained Him the victory. (Psalm 98:1 NKJV)

BREAD FOR THE SPIRIT

I love watching the championship game of any sporting event: the Super Bowl, the World Series, the Stanley Cup, the NBA Championship. I particularly like watching the members of the winning teams celebrate by dousing each other with some cold beverage. Many teams even pour a cooler of Gatorade over their coaches' heads after winning the big game. Regardless of the event, I always pay close attention to the joy and happiness that accompany winning. Today, you deserve the similar victory celebration. You have won a significant battle and have achieved the highest prize. Today, we celebrate your victory in Christ!

BREAD FOR THE SOUL

Say this prayer and write down any thoughts or requests you have for God:

Lord, I have so many things to be thankful for that it would take me a lifetime to name them all. But today, I just want to thank You for loving me enough to save me from myself. Allow me to celebrate in my own way by proudly displaying my crown of victory. Father, allow my walk with Christ to serve as a motivation and testimony for others. Amen.

BREAD FOR THE BODY

Today is your day of rest! The Lord will provide rest for your body, as well as for your soul. Enjoy the gifts of God!

Day 28	Exercises	What I Did
	Rest	
.	Read	
	Pray	

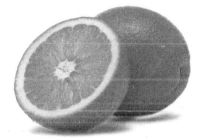

BREAD FOR THE DAY

Day 28	What to Eat	What I Ate
Breakfast	1 cup cereal	
6:30–7:30 a.m.	6 oz. low-fat milk	
	1 hard-boiled egg	
	½ cup raspberries	
Mid-morning Snack	6 wheat pretzels	
9:30–10:00 a.m.	1 plum	
Lunch	A 4-oz. turkey sub on wheat bread	
12:00–1:00 p.m.	2 celery stalks	
	1 apple	
Mid-afternoon Snack	¼ cup almonds	
3:00–3:30 p.m.	1 apple	
Dinner	An 8-oz. turkey breast	
5:30–8:00 p.m.	1 cup white rice	
	1 cup green beans	
	1 oatmeal cookie	
Calories	**1600–1800**	

Week 5

You Gotta Develop a Christian Backbone!

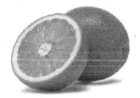

I wish I could see you right now and congratulate you in person with a big Christian hug. You have made it through four tough, transforming weeks of Christian weight loss. You are probably ready to donate your clothes to Goodwill and begin shopping for new ones. Pump your brakes for a minute. Your transformation is not yet complete. This is the last full week on your journey. We need to strengthen your framework. Within the human body, your skeletal system serves to protect your internal organs and to support your frame. It also works with your muscles to help you move. As a Christian, you also need a framework of character that protects you and helps you to move. More importantly, you need to develop a framework that keeps you from falling. This week will be dedicated to developing your Christian backbone.

It's weigh-in day again. Write down the date and your current weight below. Again, ***do not get discouraged*** by the number on your scale. Keep your mind on God and remember that it is His will, not your will. Hold on because change is coming this week!

Date: _____

Weight: _____

TESTIMONIAL

"This book has changed my life. The amazing thing is that it is so simple. I love the one-day-at-time approach. It is effective in helping you spiritually, mentally, *and* physically. I lost twenty-three pounds after my forty-day journey. This book has become a permanent part of my life, as I started all over after I completed the last step. I give all credit to the Lord and to Thomas Hundley for my success. Thank you!"

—Kathleen Nurse, Columbia, South Carolina

WEEK 5 SHOPPING LIST

List represents meal plan choices and alternatives:

Fresh Vegetables	Fresh Fruits	Canned/ Frozen	Meat	Seafood
16 servings Choose your favorites:	17 servings Choose your favorites:	• Peas • Mixed veggies • Pickles • Tomato soup • Tuna • Vegetable soup	• 6 chicken breasts • Lunch meat • Turkey bacon • Turkey breast	2 servings Choose your favorites:
• Asparagus • Broccoli • Carrots • Cauliflower • Celery • Cucumbers • Green beans • Lettuce • Peppers • Potatoes • Spinach • Sprouts • Squash • Tomatoes • Zucchini Other:	• Apples • Bananas • Blueberries • Cantaloupe • Cherries • Grapes • Kiwis • Oranges • Peaches • Pears • Plums • Raspberries • Strawberries • Tangerines Other:	Substitutes: • Applesauce • Beans • Beets • Carrots • Mixed fruit • Olives	Other:	• Crab • Flounder • Halibut • Salmon • Sardines • Scallops • Tilapia • Trout • Tuna steak Other:

Misc. Groceries	Cereal	Dairy	Breads	Snacks
	6 servings Choose your favorites:	• Eggs • Milk (1% or skim) • Sour cream • Yogurt	• Bagels • Crackers • English muffins • Whole wheat bread	• Almonds • Granola bars • Oatmeal cookies • Popcorn • Wheat pretzels • Raisins
• Baked potato chips • Chicken salad • Jelly/Jam • Natural peanut butter • Salad dressings (low-fat) • White rice • Wild rice Other:	Cold: • All-Bran • Cheerios • Granola • Grape Nuts • Life • Raisin Bran • Shredded Wheat • Special K Hot: • Cream of wheat • Grits • Kasha • Oatmeal Other:	Other:	Substitutes: • Buns • Pita bread • Rolls • Spinach wraps • Wheat wraps	Substitutes: • Cashews • Creamsicles • Dried fruit • Protein bars • Salsa • Special K bars

OBEDIENCE

Step 29

BREAD FOR THE MIND

When you become a Christian, you are tempted and tested more than ever. In those times of trial, you will need to arm yourself with God's gifts of protection. Your first step this week is to develop **obedience**. We will define *obedience* as "the active response to what God says." The Lord will make known what He expects you to do. He may instruct you through His Word, through other people, or just by telling you Himself in a quiet, gentle voice. Your obedience to God will lead to many wonderful things.

- **Obedience leads to favor.**

  If you obey me fully and keep my covenant, then out of all nations you will be my treasured possession.

  (Exodus 19:5)

- **Obedience leads to protection.**

  Everyone has heard about your obedience, so I am full of joy over you; but I want you to be wise about what is good, and innocent about what is evil. The

God of peace will soon crush Satan under your feet. (Romans 16:19–20)

- **Obedience leads others to Christ.**

Because of the service by which you have proved yourselves, men will praise God for the obedience that accompanies your confession of the gospel of Christ.
(2 Corinthians 9:13)

- **Obedience pleases God.**

By faith Abraham, when called to go to a place he would later receive as his inheritance, obeyed and went, even though he did not know where he was going. (Hebrews 11:8)

BREAD FOR THE SPIRIT
(Read 1 Kings 19:1–12)

While serving in Iraq in support of Operation Iraqi Freedom, I would occasionally escape from the chaos by working out in the gym. I purposely chose to workout at 11:00 p.m. each night to minimize my interaction with others. One day, a young, overweight airman from my Bible study class approached me. He wanted me to help him lose weight. I really did not want a workout partner infringing on my personal time of solitude, nor did I want anyone altering the pace and intensity of my workouts. In addition, the airman sometimes seemed arrogant and temperamental; he was out of shape and frequently used foul language. I prayed to God about it, and—you guessed it—God instructed me to help this young man. Out of obedience, I decided to share a lot of my precious personal time in order to help him.

On the first day of our workout, I made the airman commit to eating with me, worshipping with me, and running with me. I would occasionally catch him going to the dining facility without me, sneaking in a chili-cheese dog with fries before I arrived. What he didn't know was that God was on my side. Without fail, the Lord would allow me to catch him cheating or allow someone whom we both knew to catch him. When I caught him, I would either "strongly encourage" him to put the food back or I'd take his plate and make him watch me eat his food. That was actually quite enjoyable.

Over the course of one month, the airman lost more than twenty pounds and trimmed six inches off his waist. He accepted Christ as his personal Savior. To others, his physical, mental, and spiritual transformations were apparent. I was very proud of his physical efforts and accomplishments, but my biggest surprise was yet to come. As I entered the gym one day, I noticed several people there, each holding one of the *Purpose Driven Life* books from my Bible study class. Then, I spotted the airman carrying a camouflaged book bag and passing books out to everyone in the gym. He was starting his own crusade to bring others to Christ.

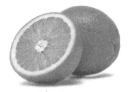

BREAD FOR THE SOUL

Say this prayer and write down any thoughts or requests you have for God:

Father, I pray for Your order of protection. Help me to build a strong Christian foundation so that I may be able to stand up during trials. I pray that You will quiet my heart so that I may hear Your instructions. Father, I pray that my faith and obedience would bring a smile to Your face and praise to Your kingdom. Amen.

BREAD FOR THE BODY

Perform thirty minutes of aerobic and anaerobic activity today. Ensure that your workout includes ten minutes of weight and strength training.

Day 29	Exercise Options	What I Did
30 minutes	Free weights	
	Strength training	
	Aerobics	
	Dumbbells	
	Resistance training	
	Fit for the King DVD	

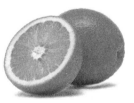

BREAD FOR THE DAY

Day 29	What to Eat	What I Ate
Breakfast	1 cup cereal	
6:30–7:30 a.m.	6 oz. low-fat milk	
	2 slices turkey bacon	
	1 apple	
Mid-morning Snack	6 crackers w/ jam	
9:30–10:00 a.m.	1 pear	
Lunch	A 4-oz. turkey sandwich on wheat w/ low-fat dressing	
12:00–1:00 p.m.	½ cup vegetable soup	
Mid-afternoon Snack	½ bagel	
3:00–3:30 p.m.	1 Tbsp. jelly	
Dinner	4 oz. grilled chicken breast	
5:30–8:00 p.m.	1 cup wild rice	
	1 cup green beans	
Calories	**1500–1800**	

COMPASSION

Step 30

BREAD FOR THE MIND

God shows His love for you through His gifts of grace and mercy. As a Christian, you are expected to show love for others by giving them the gift of **compassion**. We will define *compassion* as "the active display of concern for others." The next step on your journey is to build compassion. Here are some biblical examples:

- **Compassion shows mercy.**

  The LORD is gracious and compassionate, slow to anger and rich in love. (Psalm 145:8)

- **Compassion influences others in positive ways.**

  Jesus had compassion on them and touched their eyes. Immediately they received their sight and followed him. (Matthew 20:34)

- **Compassion strengthens.**

  He can have compassion on those who are ignorant

and going astray, since he himself is also subject to weakness. (Hebrews 5:2 NKJV)

- Compassion shows love.

Finally, all of you, live in harmony with one another; be sympathetic, love as brothers, be compassionate and humble. (1 Peter 3:8)

BREAD FOR THE SPIRIT
(Read Luke 10:25–37)

One of the greatest stories in the Bible is that of the Good Samaritan. It contains many teaching points that are applicable today. How many times have you seen someone stranded along the road, yet you did not stop to help him or her? How many people have you known to need assistance, yet you looked the other way?

In the story of the Good Samaritan, even a priest passed by the beaten man without offering help. It turns out that none of us is perfect; we all have room for improvement. I am convinced that the world is full of Good Samaritans. I have seen the generous donations that my fellow Americans contributed to victims of Hurricane Katrina. I have seen the kind and compassionate people who quit their jobs to serve as volunteers to rebuild and restore New Orleans. God wants you to develop a strong sense of compassion for others. The Lord is showing you compassion by transforming your body. You have an opportunity to show your love and compassion for others by sharing the Good News. Today, share your story with someone else.

BREAD FOR THE SOUL

Say this prayer and write down any thoughts or requests you have for God:

Father in heaven, I want to thank You for having mercy on my soul. Thank You for giving me biblical examples of how to show compassion. I pray that You would place someone in my path today who needs to experience Your compassion. Allow me to use my struggles, my trials, and my experience to influence someone to want to know You. Amen.

BREAD FOR THE BODY

Perform thirty minutes of aerobic and anaerobic exercise today. Your workout session should target toning your lower body with emphasis on the thighs, hips, and buttocks.

Day 30	Exercise Options	What I Did
30 minutes	Free weights	
	Strength training	
	Aerobics	
	Dumbbells	
	Resistance training	
	Fit for the King DVD	

BREAD FOR THE DAY

Day 30	What to Eat	What I Ate
Breakfast	1 cup cereal	
6:30–7:30 a.m.	6 oz. low-fat milk	
	1 oz. raisins	
	1 slice toast w/ 1 Tbsp. jam	
Mid-morning Snack	1 granola bar	
9:30–10:00 a.m.	1 banana	
Lunch	A 4-oz. turkey sandwich with lettuce and tomato	
12:00–1:00 p.m.	1 oz. baked potato chips	
Mid-afternoon Snack	4 wheat pretzels	
3:00–3:30 p.m.	6 strawberries	
Dinner	6 oz. baked fish	
5:30–8:00 p.m.	1 cup broccoli	
	1 baked potato	
	1 Tbsp. sour cream	
Calories	**1500–1800**	

HUMILITY

Step 31

BREAD FOR THE MIND

Being a follower of Christ means you must develop an attitude like Christ. One thing your attitude must contain is the motto, "It's not about me." The next step on your weight loss journey is to develop **humility**. We will define *humility* as "the active praise and recognition of others over your own worth." This step requires you to give God the credit for everything you accomplish, experience, and overcome. You must realize that God is our Creator and Redeemer; without Him, we are worthless. This realization will lead you to develop the Christlike characteristic of humility.

- **Glorify Jesus, not yourself.**

  I am the vine; you are the branches. If a man remains in me and I in him, he will bear much fruit; apart from me you can do nothing. (John 15:5)

- **Honor God, not yourself.**

  For by the grace given me I say to every one of you:

do not think of yourself more highly than you ought, but rather think of yourself with sober judgment, in accordance with the measure of faith God has given you. (Romans 12:3)

- **Credit God, not yourself.**

For it is by grace you have been saved, through faith— and this not from yourselves, it is the gift of God. (Ephesians 2:8)

- **Compliment others, not yourself**

Do nothing out of selfish ambition or vain conceit, but in humility consider others better than yourselves. (Philippians 2:3)

- **Serve God, not yourself.**

The Lord's servant must not quarrel; instead, he must be kind to everyone, able to teach, not resentful. Those who oppose him he must gently instruct, in the hope that God will grant them repentance leading them to a knowledge of the truth. (2 Timothy 2:24–25)

BREAD FOR THE SPIRIT
(Read Matthew 20:20–28)

Humility is one of my favorite topics of debate. I am always fascinated by people who seem to think more highly of themselves than they ought. You see this behavior in the professional athlete who boasts about his performance and abilities as though he invented them himself. You see it in the radio talk show personality who demeans others as if he or she is without blemish or fault. You see it in the academic scholar who believes superior education makes him or her more intelligent than God. Then there is the heir or heiress of a wealthy family whose arrogance is predicated on the accomplishments of his or her parents.

My overall favorite, however, are the arrogant Christians who boast about their Christianity as if they are the only ones in the world whom God has saved. They act as if they are without sin. They articulate God's Word with such anger and malice that it demeans and judges others rather than edifying them. I submit to all of those who fall into this category, *It's not about you.* You are significant only because God chose to make you significant. Remember, even Jesus was sent here to serve others and not Himself. (See Mark 10:45.) Recall that even Jesus humbled Himself by washing the feet of others. (See John 13:5.) To understand fully what it means to be humble, you are not even allowed to list humility as one of your characteristics. Give God the praise for your accomplishments today and remember, *it's not about you.*

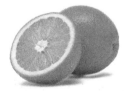

BREAD FOR THE SOUL

Say this prayer and write down any thoughts or requests you have for God:

Lord, today I want to give You all of the glory, honor, and praise for all the blessings you have provided. I realize that I am nothing without You. I recognize Your presence in my life and know that by Your grace and mercy, I am saved. Father, I pray that You would continue to develop Christlike characteristics within me. Amen.

BREAD FOR THE BODY

Perform thirty minutes of cardiorespiratory and/or aerobic activity.

Day 31	Exercise Options	What I Did
30 minutes	Walk	
	Run	
	Treadmill	
	Aerobics	
	Elliptical machine	
	Bicycle	
	Fit for the King DVD	

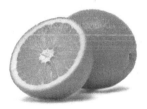

BREAD FOR THE DAY

Day 31	What to Eat	What I Ate
Breakfast	1 cup oatmeal	
6:30–7:30 a.m.	6 oz. low-fat milk	
	2 slices turkey bacon	
	½ grapefruit	
Mid-morning Snack	6 baby carrot sticks	
9:30–10:00 a.m.	1 Tbsp. low-fat dressing	
Lunch	1 peanut butter & jelly sandwich	
12:00–1:00 p.m.	1 orange	
Mid-afternoon Snack	1 granola bar	
3:00–3:30 p.m.	1 peach	
Dinner	4 oz. grilled salmon	
5:30–8:00 p.m.	1 cup green beans	
	1 baked potato	
	1 Tbsp. sour cream	
Calories	**1300–1600**	

KINDNESS

Step 32

BREAD FOR THE MIND

With each passing day, you are developing more and more Christlike characteristics. You are also developing a body that will stand during the trials and tribulations that life brings. The next step on your Christian weight loss journey is to develop **kindness.** We will define *kindness* as "the active display of love and generosity toward others." God shows His loving-kindness to us through His grace and mercy. He graciously forgives us and mercifully keeps His promises to His chosen people despite our sinful natures. Because God has been so loving and kind to us, He expects us to show the same love and kindness to others.

- **Be kind to your enemies.**

Love your enemies, do good to them, and lend to them without expecting to get anything back. Then your reward will be great, and you will be sons of the Most High, because he is kind to the ungrateful and wicked. (Luke 6:35)

- **Be kind in correction.**

The Lord's servant must not quarrel; instead, he must be kind to everyone, able to teach, not resentful. Those who oppose him he must gently instruct, in the hope that God will grant them repentance leading them to a knowledge of the truth.

(2 Timothy 2:24–25)

- **Be kind in forgiveness.**

Be kind and compassionate to one another, forgiving each other, just as in Christ God forgave you.

(Ephesians 4:32)

- **Be kind for salvation.**

But the fruit of the Spirit is love, joy, peace, patience, kindness, goodness, faithfulness, gentleness and self-control. Against such things there is no law.

(Galatians 5:22)

BREAD FOR THE SPIRIT

One of my good Christian friends has been participating in a homeless ministry for her church. She shared with me how she met a homeless couple who did not believe in God. Despite their beliefs, she continued to provide them with spiritual encouragement by telling them about the goodness of God. She would routinely pray for them in their presence and ask God to bless them and their situation. After about three months of seemingly unanswered prayers, my friend began to feel frustration and doubt. She immediately changed the way she prayed by expressing her frustration to the Lord. As she prayed, she said, "Okay, Lord. I have these people here who need to know how wonderful You are. How can I get them to pray to You when my prayers seem to go unanswered? I know that everything happens in Your timing and in Your will, but I am asking you for a miracle. You said that anything I ask in Jesus' name will be granted unto me. I am asking You in the name of Jesus to bless this couple so that they may believe in Your greatness. Amen."

Within three days of that prayer, a couple anonymously donated one of their homes to the ministry. Not only did the homeless couple have a new place to live, but they were also given full ownership of the home. They are now members of a church and have accepted Christ as their personal Savior. It is simply amazing what a little kindness, love, and prayer can do to change a heart. Show Christlike kindness to someone you meet today.

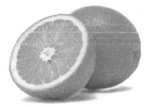

BREAD FOR THE SOUL

Say this prayer and write down any thoughts or requests you have for God:

Dear heavenly Father, I strive each day to become more like Your Son, Jesus. I realize that there are things within me that I must change. I pray for Your help and guidance in making me a more kind and gentle soul. Lord, today I ask that You would give me a prime opportunity to show kindness to others. Amen.

BREAD FOR THE BODY

Perform thirty minutes of aerobic and anaerobic activity today. Ensure that your workout includes ten minutes of weight and strength training.

Day 32	Exercise Options	What I Did
30 minutes	Free weights	
	Strength training	
	Aerobics	
	Dumbbells	
	Resistance training	
	Fit for the King DVD	

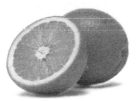

BREAD FOR THE DAY

Day 32	What to Eat	What I Ate
Breakfast 6:30–7:30 a.m.	1 English muffin with jam ½ cup granola 1 banana	
Mid-morning Snack 9:30–10:00 a.m.	1 granola bar 1 plum	
Lunch 12:00–1:00 p.m.	A 4-oz. tuna sandwich on wheat on wheat bread 1 Tbsp. low-fat dressing 2 celery stalks	
Mid-afternoon Snack 3:00–3:30 p.m.	¼ cup almonds 1 pear	
Dinner 5:30–8:00 p.m.	6 oz. baked chicken 1 cup wild rice ½ cup carrots ½ cup peas	
Calories	**1400–1700**	

FRIENDSHIP

Step 33

BREAD FOR THE MIND

God deeply desires for us to get to know Him personally and intimately. You have already mastered many of the steps required to know God on a personal level. God requires that you read and meditate on His Word, pray and communicate with Him daily, and obey His commands. Your next step on this journey requires you to develop a closer **friendship** with God. We will define *friendship* as "the active companionship and bonding with another."

- **Your friendship with God requires obedience.**

  You are my friends if you do what I command.

  (John 15:14)

- **Your friendship with God provides protection.**

  Though I walk in the midst of trouble, you preserve my life; you stretch out your hand against the anger of my foes, with your right hand you save me.

  (Psalm 138:77)

- **Your friendship with God requires passion.**

I want to know Christ and the power of his resurrection and the fellowship of sharing in his sufferings, becoming like him in his death. (Philippians 3:10)

- **Your friendship with God provides freedom.**

I no longer call you servants, because a servant does not know his master's business. Instead, I have called you friends, for everything that I learned from my Father I have made known to you. (John 15:15)

BREAD FOR THE SPIRIT
(Read John 15:12–17)

The Bible provides a perfect illustration of friendship. In 1 Samuel 18, we find the story of David and Jonathan. Their friendship was more than just mere companionship. The Bible mentions that their souls were connected. Their friendship was so strong that they made a covenant with one another. Jonathan loved David as strongly as he loved himself. True friendship requires that you show love. The best example of the depth of that love can also be found in John 15:13, which states, *"Greater love has no one than this, that he lay down his life for his friends."* Today is the day for you to seek a closer relationship with Jesus. This is your gateway to a life of protection and blessing.

BREAD FOR THE SOUL

Say this prayer and write down any thoughts or requests you have for God:

Father, forgive me for being too busy to establish a closer relationship with You. I know that in order to become Your close friend, I must pray to You continuously. I know that I must read and meditate on Your Word daily. Finally, I know that I must obey Your commands and desire You above all else. Lord, help me to remind myself to talk to You more often each day. Amen.

BREAD FOR THE BODY

Perform thirty minutes of aerobic and anaerobic activity today. Ensure that your workout includes ten minutes of weight and strength training.

Day 33	Exercise Options	What I Did
30 minutes	Free weights	
	Strength training	
	Aerobics	
	Dumbbells	
	Resistance training	
	Fit for the King DVD	

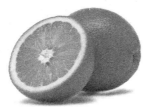

BREAD FOR THE DAY

Day 33	What to Eat	What I Ate
Breakfast	1 cup cereal	
6:30–7:30 a.m.	6 oz. low-fat milk	
	½ cup raisins	
Mid-morning Snack	2 celery stalks	
9:30–10:00 a.m.	1 Tbsp. natural peanut butter	
Lunch	A 4-oz. turkey sandwich on wheat bread w/ lettuce, tomato, and pickle	
12:00–1:00 p.m.	½ cup tomato soup	
	1 apple	
Mid-afternoon Snack	¼ cup almonds	
3:00–3:30 p.m.	1 orange	
Dinner	6 oz. BBQ chicken breast	
5:30–8:00 p.m.	1 cup wild rice	
	1 cup vegetable	
Calories	**1200–1600**	

Struggle

Step 34

Bread for the Mind

If God really loves us, then why does He allow so much pain and suffering in the world? The life of a Christian is not always easy. We live in a world cursed with sin. As part of the growth and development on your Christian journey, you will face trials and sufferings that will serve a far greater purpose. We will refer to these trials as **struggle** and define *struggle* as "the active suffering and testing of Christians used by God as an educational tool." This is how God uses struggle in our lives:

- **To Teach Us Obedience**

  It was good for me to suffer so I would learn your demands. (Psalm 119:71 NCV)

- **To Test Our Faith**

  Examine yourselves to see whether you are in the

faith; test yourselves. Do you not realize that Christ Jesus is in you—unless, of course, you fail the test?
(2 Corinthians 13:5)

• To Shape Us

For our light and momentary troubles are achieving for us an eternal glory that far outweighs them all.
(2 Corinthians 4:17)

• To Awaken Compassion in Us

Praise be to the God and Father of our Lord Jesus Christ, the Father of compassion and the God of all comfort, who comforts us in all our troubles, so that we can comfort those in any trouble with the comfort we ourselves have received from God.
(2 Corinthians 1:3–4)

• To Keep Us Humble

I am in prison because I belong to the Lord. Therefore I urge you who have been chosen by God to live up to the life to which God called you. Always be humble, gentle, and patient, accepting each other in love.
(Ephesians 4:1–2 NCV)

• To Make Us More Like Christ

Dear friends, do not be surprised at the painful trial you are suffering, as though something strange were happening to you. But rejoice that you participate in the sufferings of Christ, so that you may be overjoyed when his glory is revealed.   (1 Peter 4:12–13)

Bread for the Spirit:
(Read Job 1–2)

Today is the most important education lesson on your Christian weight loss journey. To be a disciple of Christ, you will have to suffer like Christ. Mel Gibson made the *Oscar*-nominated movie *The Passion of the Christ*. I was reluctant to watch the movie at first, but I am so glad that I did. After watching it, I was able to comprehend more fully the sufferings Jesus had to endure. I asked myself, *Would I have sacrificed my life for the same purpose?* When I compared my meager problems and situations to those of Jesus, I was embarrassed. Now, when I go through those rough patches that life throws my way, I reflect back on the sufferings of Jesus. I find joy and comfort knowing that my momentary troubles pale in comparison to the One who died for me.

Don't be afraid of the trials and suffering that you must endure. God reminds us, *"My grace is sufficient for you, for my power is made perfect in weakness"* (2 Corinthians 12:9). In fact, you should actually smile and rejoice when you struggle, for the Lord will test those whom He has personally chosen to do His work. That makes *you* someone special! So, when you find yourself going through trying times, heartache, and pain, reflect on the sufferings of Christ. Remember the sufferings of Job. Compare your situation to theirs. Would you like to trade places with them?

BREAD FOR THE SOUL

Say this prayer and write down any thoughts or requests you have for God:

Father God, I pray for Your grace and mercy during my trials and tribulations. Help me to remember that my suffering is only temporary. Help me to understand the purpose of my struggle. I pray that I might be able to use my experiences and sufferings to help someone else during similar trials. Lord, I pray that others will see Your strength in my weakness. Amen.

BREAD FOR THE BODY

Perform thirty minutes of aerobic and anaerobic exercise today. Your workout session should target toning your lower body with emphasis on the thighs, hips, and buttocks.

Day 34	Exercise Options	What I Did
30 minutes	Free weights	
	Strength training	
	Aerobics	
	Dumbbells	
	Resistance training	
	Fit for the King DVD	

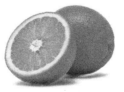

BREAD FOR THE DAY

Day 34	What to Eat	What I Ate
Breakfast	1 cup cereal	
6:30–7:30 a.m.	6 oz. low-fat milk	
	1 hard-boiled egg	
	½ cup raspberries	
Mid-morning Snack	2 cups popcorn	
9:30–10:00 a.m.	1 plum	
Lunch	A 4-oz. turkey sub on wheat bread	
12:00–1:00 p.m.	1 Tbsp. low-fat dressing	
	2 celery stalks	
Mid-afternoon Snack	¼ cup almonds	
3:00–3:30 p.m.	1 apple	
Dinner	8 oz. turkey breast	
5:30–8:00 p.m.	1 cup broccoli	
	½ cup white rice	
	1 oatmeal cookie	
Calories	**1300–1600**	

Step 35

BREAD FOR THE MIND

The final step in building your Christian backbone is to develop and strengthen your **Christianity**. We will define *Christianity* as "the active belief in the birth, life, death, and resurrection of Jesus Christ." Christianity is more than just a religion or belief system. For those who choose to follow Christ, Christianity is a way of life. By accepting Christ as your personal Savior, you become members of His body—the church. Here are the privileges that come with your membership:

- **Salvation**

  Salvation is found in no one else, for there is no other name under heaven given to men by which we must be saved. (Acts 4:12)

- **Justification**

  Know that a man is not justified by observing the law, but by faith in Jesus Christ. So we, too, have put our faith in Christ Jesus that we may be justified by faith in Christ and not by observing the law, because by observing the law no one will be justified.

(Galatians 2:16)

- **Christlikeness**

And we, who with unveiled faces all reflect the Lord's glory, are being transformed into his likeness with ever-increasing glory, which comes from the Lord, who is the Spirit. (2 Corinthians 3:18)

- **Righteousness**

However, if you suffer as a Christian, do not be ashamed, but praise God that you bear that name.

(1 Peter 4:16)

BREAD FOR THE SPIRIT

You should strive to strengthen your Christianity around the principle that Jesus Christ is the only Savior and the sole gateway between God and mankind. **Warning:** Please do not attempt to use your membership in a manner that separates, segregates, or divides you from other people. Your behavior should *never* reflect that of one who is pompous, arrogant, or conceited. Believe it or not, there are some Christians who behave in this manner. Remember to always practice compassion, humility, and kindness. (See Steps 31, 32, and 33.)

BREAD FOR THE SOUL:

Say this prayer and write down any thoughts or requests you have for God:

Father, give me a clear conscience and clean heart to be a unifier and not a divider. Help me practice humility, kindness, and compassion today so that I may connect with other believers and nonbelievers. Lord, please give the wisdom and understanding I need to make a difference in this world. Amen.

_____

_____

_____

_____

_____

_____

_____

_____

_____

_____

_____

_____

_____

BREAD FOR THE BODY

Today is your day of rest! Reflect on your Christian growth and development.

Day 35	Exercise Options	What I Did
	Rest	
	Read	
	Pray	

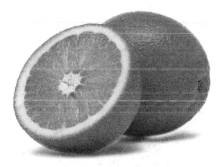

BREAD FOR THE DAY

Day 35	What to Eat	What I Ate
Breakfast	1 English muffin with jam	
6:30–7:30 a.m.	1 hard-boiled egg	
	1 banana	
Mid-morning Snack	1 granola bar	
9:30–10:00 a.m.	1 plum	
Lunch	A 4-oz. tuna sandwich on wheat bread	
12:00–1:00 p.m.	1 Tbsp. low-fat dressing	
	2 celery stalks	
Mid-afternoon Snack	¼ cup almonds	
3:00–3:30 p.m.	1 pear	
Dinner	6 oz. baked chicken	
5:30–8:00 p.m.	½ cup wild rice	
	½ cup carrots	
	½ cup vegetables	
Calories	**1300–1600**	

Week 6

You Gotta Know How to Work It!

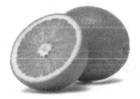

You are in the home stretch! You have successfully completed your fifth week of Christian weight loss. Are you ready for that new wardrobe yet? You have probably noticed some positive physical changes in your body. If so, take a moment to celebrate by giving God the praise.

The Lord has shaped and prepared you spiritually and physically for a specific mission. You have five more days to go, and these days are critical. The Lord will speak to you during this week, so it is important for you to open your heart and mind to hear His voice. The next five days will be devoted to learning how to use the gifts that God has given you. Each of your next five steps will require that you reflect on the things that you learned along your journey.

It's weigh-in day again. Write down the date and your current weight below. Keep your mind on God and remember that it is His will, not your will. Hold on because your revelation is coming!

Date: _____

Weight: _____

WEEK 6 SHOPPING LIST

List represents meal plan choices and alternatives:

Fresh Vegetables	Fresh Fruits	Canned/ Frozen	Meat	Seafood
12 servings Choose your favorites:	6 servings Choose your favorites:	• Tuna • Vegetable soup	• 2 chicken breasts • Ground turkey • Lunch meat • Turkey bacon	3 servings Choose your favorites:
• Asparagus • Broccoli • Carrots • Cauliflower • Celery • Cucumbers • Green beans • Lettuce • Peppers • Potatoes • Spinach • Sprouts • Squash • Tomatoes • Zucchini Other:	• Apples • Bananas • Blueberries • Cantaloupe • Cherries • Grapes • Kiwis • Oranges • Peaches • Pears • Plums • Raspberries • Strawberries • Tangerines Other:	Substitutes: • Applesauce • Beans • Beets • Carrots • Peas • Mixed fruit • Mixed veggies • Olives • Pasta sauce • Pickles • Soups • Tomatoes	Other:	• Crab • Flounder • Halibut • Salmon • Sardines • Scallops • Tilapia • Trout • Tuna steak Other:

Misc. Groceries	Cereal	Dairy	Breads	Snacks
• Jelly/Jam • Natural peanut butter • Salad dressings (low-fat) • White rice • Wild rice Other:	3 servings Choose your favorites: Cold: • All-Bran • Cheerios • Granola • Grape Nuts • Life • Raisin Bran • Shredded Wheat • Special K Hot: • Cream of wheat • Grits • Oatmeal Other:	• Eggs • Milk (1% or Skim) • Yogurt Other:	• Crackers • English muffins • Whole wheat bread • Rolls • Spinach wraps Substitutes: • Bagels • Buns • Pita bread • Wheat wraps	• Almonds • Creamsicles • Salsa Substitutes: • Cashews • Dried fruit • Granola bars • Multigrain chips • Oatmeal cookies • Popcorn • Pretzels • Protein bars • Raisins • Special K bars

Step 36

BREAD FOR THE MIND

God loves you, and He is smiling on you right now. The fact that you have made it this far in your journey truly pleases Him. When you do things that bring pleasure to God, you are performing acts of **worship**. We will define *worship* as "physical and spiritual acts of devotion and allegiance to God." Your next step requires that you live a life that pleases God. This is what you can do to make God smile through worship:

- **Give God your love (Step 3).**

  "Love the Lord your God with all your heart and with all your soul and with all your mind." This is the first and greatest commandment.

  (Matthew 22:37–38)

- **Give God your trust (Step 6).**

  Blessed is the man who trusts in the LORD, whose confidence is in him. (Jeremiah 17:7)

- **Give God your body (Step 7).**

I urge you, brothers, in view of God's mercy, to offer your bodies as living sacrifices, holy and pleasing to God—this is your spiritual act of worship.
(Romans 12:1)

- **Give God your praises (Step 13).**

It is good to praise the LORD and make music to your name, O Most High. (Psalm 92:1)

- **Give God your obedience (Step 29).**

Now if you obey me fully and keep my covenant, then out of all nations you will be my treasured possession. (Exodus 19:5)

BREAD FOR THE SPIRIT
(Read John 4:7–24)

Everything you have belongs to God. He gave you many possessions so that He may delight in your enjoyment of those possessions. When you properly care for His possessions, He smiles on you and gives you even more. But don't take my word for it; I give you God's Word: Luke 16:10, where Jesus said, *"Whoever can be trusted with very little can also be trusted with much, and whoever is dishonest with very little will also be dishonest with much."* Here are a few areas in your life in which you can worship God:

- **Your body.** (See 1 Corinthians 6:19–20.)
- **Your talents and abilities.** (See Psalm 37:23.)

- **Your words.** (See Hebrews 13:15.)
- **Your lifestyle.** (See James 2:24.)
- **Your material possessions.** (See 1 Timothy 6:17.)
- **Your eating habits.** (See 1 Corinthians 10:31.)

Worship requires you to get in the game and participate. You can no longer sit on the bench and think that God is pleased just because you are a member of the team. From this day forward, you must always remember that you were not created to please only yourself. You were created for *God's* pleasure. When you devote your life to pleasing Him, He will return the favor ten times over. God is smiling on you right now. Start your day with a small act of worship. Look up to the heavens and say, "Thank You, Lord!"

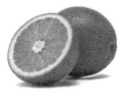

BREAD FOR THE SOUL

Say this prayer and write down any thoughts or requests you have for God:

Father, I thank You for smiling on me today. Today, I want to dedicate and devote my entire life to pleasing You. Help me to trust You, to obey You, and to love You with all that I have. Lord, help me to properly care for all of the things that You have given me. I pray that everything I do, everything I say, and everything I think would be holy and pleasing to You. Empower me with a lifestyle of worship. Amen.

BREAD FOR THE BODY

Perform thirty minutes of aerobic and anaerobic activity today. Ensure that your workout includes ten minutes of weight and strength training.

Day 36	Exercise Options	What I Did
30 minutes	Free weights	
	Strength training	
	Aerobics	
	Dumbbells	
	Resistance training	
	Fit for the King DVD	

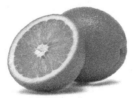

BREAD FOR THE DAY

Day 36	What to Eat	What I Ate
Breakfast	1 cup oatmeal	
6:30–7:30 a.m.	6 oz. low-fat milk	
	2 slices turkey bacon	
	1 apple	
Mid-morning Snack	6 crackers with jam	
9:30–10:00 a.m.	1 pear	
Lunch	A 4-oz. roast beef sandwich on wheat bread	
12:00–1:00 p.m.	1 Tbsp. low-fat dressing	
	½ cup vegetable soup	
Mid-afternoon Snack	½ English muffin	
3:00–3:30 p.m.	1 Tbsp. jelly	
Dinner	4 oz. grilled chicken	
5:30–8:00 p.m.	1 cup wild rice	
	1 cup green beans	
	1 apple	
Calories	**1500–1800**	

FELLOWSHIP

Step 37

BREAD FOR THE MIND

We live in a world with more than one billion other people. God did not create all of us to keep to ourselves. Each one of us is given a unique path to follow. On our paths, we all have gained certain levels of knowledge and encountered a certain number of experiences. God intends for us to bring our individuality into a collective forum. He intends for us to share ourselves openly with others so that we can continue to grow spiritually. The Lord calls this collective sharing of knowledge and experiences **fellowship.** For a more accurate definition, we will define *fellowship* as "the active sharing of commonalities and differences with others." Here are five steps to developing productive Christian fellowship:

- **Put God first.**

  God, who has called you into fellowship with his Son Jesus Christ our Lord, is faithful.

  (1 Corinthians 1:9)

- **Come together in Christ.**

  But if we walk in the light, as he is in the light, we have fellowship with one another, and the blood of Jesus, his Son, purifies us from all sin. (1 John 1:7)

- **Bring love to the party.**

  A new command I give you: Love one another. As I have loved you, so you must love one another.
  (John 13:34)

- **Pursue peaceful unions.**

  Let us therefore make every effort to do what leads to peace and to mutual edification. (Romans 14:19)

- **Be the peacemaker.**

  Now the fruit of righteousness is sown in peace by those who make peace. (James 3:18 NKJV)

BREAD FOR THE SPIRIT
(Read Romans 12:9–18)

Building genuine fellowship with other Christians takes a multitude of Christlike characteristics. These are characteristics that you now possess as a result of taking this journey, and they include:

- **Love** (Step 3)
- **Compassion** (Step 30)
- **Humility** (Step 31)
- **Kindness** (Step 32)
- **Friendship** (Step 33)

When you come together as a group of individuals, you are assured to have many differences. It is important that you *do not* focus on your differences, but that you focus instead on the one thing you all have in common: Christ Jesus. When you develop genuine fellowship with a like-minded group of believers, you form a family connection. In this family, you feel comfortable sharing your deepest feelings, thoughts, and fears with others who may have already experienced something similar to your current situation. God smiles on genuine fellowship. He stands by, waiting for you to share yourself openly with others. He stands by, watching as you show sympathy and compassion for others. Then, when you collectively call on Him for help, He stands by, mercifully waiting to answer your call. Remember, God said in His Word, *"Where two or three come together in my name, there am I with them"* (Matthew 18:20). Pursue fellowship with a group of Christians today.

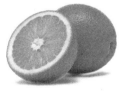

BREAD FOR THE SOUL:

Say this prayer and write down any thoughts or requests you have for God:

Father God, I realize that I need others in my life in order for me to grow spiritually. I understand that You did not place me on earth to be alone. Help me to develop strong fellowship with other Christians so I may openly experience the kingdom of God and share your Good News. Heavenly Father, I ask that You would give me many opportunities to develop my Christlike characteristics of love, humility, compassion, kindness, and friendship. Amen.

BREAD FOR THE BODY

Perform thirty minutes of aerobic and anaerobic exercise today. Your workout session should target toning your lower body with emphasis on the thighs, hips, and buttocks.

Day 37	Exercise Options	What I Did
30 minutes	Free weights	
	Strength training	
	Aerobics	
	Dumbbells	
	Resistance training	
	Fit for the King DVD	

BREAD FOR THE DAY

Day 37	What to Eat	What I Ate
Breakfast	1 slice of toast w/ jam	
6:30–7:30 a.m.	½ cup yogurt w/ granola	
	1 orange	
Mid-morning Snack	½ English muffin	
9:30–10:00 a.m.	1 Tbsp. jelly	
Lunch	A 4-oz. tuna salad sandwich	
12:00–1:00 p.m.	1 Tbsp. low-fat dressing	
	2 celery stalks	
Mid-afternoon Snack	6 crackers w/ jam	
3:00–3:30 p.m.	1 pear	
Dinner	6 oz. grilled salmon	
5:30–8:00 p.m.	1 cup wild rice	
	½ cup carrots	
	½ cup green beans	
Calories	**1400–1700**	

Step 38

BREAD FOR THE MIND

The next step on your Christian weight loss journey is to learn about the joy of **giving.** We will define *giving* as "the act of providing someone with something without expecting anything in return." God is the giver of every good and perfect gift. (See James 1:17.) These gifts include salvation, eternal life, food, physical attributes, spiritual abilities, and the greatest gift of all: His Son, Jesus Christ. The Lord commands that we give from our hearts and not out of compulsion. Here are four steps that I use when it comes to giving:

- **Give to those in need.**

  There will always be poor people in the land. Therefore I command you to be openhanded toward your brothers and toward the poor and needy in your land. (Deuteronomy 15:11)

- **Give of yourself with good deeds.**

  Command them to do good, to be rich in good deeds, and to be generous and willing to share.

  (1 Timothy 6:18)

- **Give generously of your blessings.**

Remember this: Whoever sows sparingly will also reap sparingly, and whoever sows generously will also reap generously. (2 Corinthians 9:6)

- **Give to be blessed abundantly.**

Give, and it will be given to you. A good measure, pressed down, shaken together and running over, will be poured into your lap. For with the measure you use, it will be measured to you. (Luke 6:38)

BREAD FOR THE SPIRIT
(Read 2 Corinthians 9:6–11)

This entire Christian weight loss journey has been full of giving and receiving. You gave up man's methods of weight loss; you received God's perfect method of weight loss. You gave your body and your time to Christ; you received a slimmer physique and a healthier lifestyle. Over the past five weeks, you have practiced and perfected the art of giving through your various steps. Let's reflect:

- **You gave Jesus your love and devotion.** (Step 3)

- **You gave your life to Christ.** (Step 7)

- **You gave God the credit for your achievements.** (Step 13)

- **You gave your word that you will serve the Lord.** (Step 21)

- **You gave your sympathetic ear to someone in need.** (Step 30)

The Lord is truly pleased with your accomplishments. He has already rewarded you with His good and perfect gifts. (See Steps 22–28.) Now, it is time for you to give to others so that they may understand the art of giving. Take a moment of your time today to bless someone else as the Lord has blessed you. There is no greater feeling than knowing that someone else may benefit greatly from your generosity. Be of good cheer and give out of the abundance of your heart. Always remember, *"God loves a cheerful giver"* (2 Corinthians 9:7).

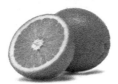

BREAD FOR THE SOUL

Say this prayer and write down any thoughts or requests you have for God:

Blessed Savior, I want to thank You for all of the blessings You have bestowed on me. I want to thank You for loving me so much that You gave Your only begotten Son to die for my sins. Teach me how to give without expecting compensation and to give without reluctance. I pray that You might bring someone into my life today whom I may bless with an act of generosity. Amen.

_____

_____

_____

_____

_____

_____

_____

_____

_____

_____

_____

BREAD FOR THE BODY

Perform thirty minutes of cardiorespiratory and/or aerobic activity.

Day 38	Exercise Options	What I Did
30 minutes	Walk	
	Run	
	Treadmill	
	Aerobics	
	Elliptical machine	
	Bicycle	
	Fit for the King DVD	

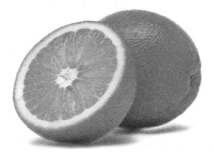

BREAD FOR THE DAY

Day 38	What to Eat	What I Ate
Breakfast 6:30–7:30 a.m.	Fast and pray	Do not eat anything
Mid-morning Snack 9:30–10:00 a.m.	Fast and pray	Do not eat anything
Lunch 12:00–1:00 p.m.	A 4-oz. grilled chicken wrap / 1 Tbsp. low-fat dressing / 6 baby carrots	
Mid-afternoon Snack 3:00–3:30 p.m.	2 celery stalks / 1 Tbsp. natural peanut butter	
Dinner 5:30–8:00 p.m.	A 6-oz. turkey burger / 1 cup white rice / 1 cup broccoli / 1 whole wheat bun	
Calories	**1000–1400**	

WITNESS

Step 39

BREAD FOR THE MIND

Now that you know how to fellowship with others and give to others, you are ready to be a **witness**. The word *witness* has several meanings, but for your Christian weight loss purposes, we are going to use three definitions. We will define *witness* (noun) as "a person who gives a firsthand account of something seen, heard, or experienced." *Witness* (verb) is defined as "to give truthful testimony." There is a third definition of witness that I believe is vitally important, too. Before you can actually *be* a witness or *do* the act of witnessing, you must be able to *see* something. So, we will also define *witness* (verb) as "to observe something." It is your duty to go out and tell the world about the things God has done for you. Here's how you can witness for Christ:

- **Witness by being.**

  You will be my witnesses. (Acts 1:8)

  Be diligent in these matters; give yourself wholly to them, so that everyone may see your progress.
  (1 Timothy 4:15)

- **Witness by doing.**

I have testimony weightier than that of John. For the very work that the Father has given me to finish, and which I am doing, testifies that the Father has sent me. (John 5:36)

- **Witness by speaking.**

I will praise you, O LORD, with all my heart; I will tell of all your wonders. (Psalm 9:1)

- **Witness by seeing.**

He came as a witness to testify concerning that light, so that through him all men might believe. He himself was not the light; he came only as a witness to the light. (John 1:7–8)

I have seen and I testify that this is the Son of God. (John 1:34)

BREAD FOR THE SPIRIT
(Read Matthew 9:1–8)

Be a witness! It amazes me that it took me thirty-two years to understand what that really meant. Surprisingly, I did not receive my revelation through a biblical or spiritual encounter. Instead, I was inspired by the hundreds of signs and billboards posted by Cleveland Cavalier fans in reference to LeBron James. Watching LeBron play a game of basketball is an unparalleled experience. Never in my life have I seen someone so young possess the phenomenal natural ability of this young athlete. After I first watched him play, all I wanted to do was tell people about what I had seen and experienced. It was at that time that the simple but emphatic message, "Be a Witness," made perfect sense.

The Lord wants you to be a witness for Him. Within approximately six weeks, the Lord has personally transformed you into a new person. He has given you all the tools you need to serve as His messenger:

- **God has given you a heart of love.** (Step 3)
- **God has given you something to be passionate about.** (Step 10)
- **God has given you the energy needed to endure.** (Step 16)
- **God has taken away all of your fears.** (Step 18)
- **God has given you the ability to walk with your head high.** (Step 19)

You now have a new lifestyle. You have new energy. You own a new body. More importantly, God has given you His love and salvation. Now, He wants you to tell others about your journey. He wants you to stand up and testify on His behalf. You have already *seen* the miracles that God can perform. There are millions of people out there who don't know the greatness of God. You have the opportunity to change—and possibly save—a person's life just by sharing the things you have experienced. Today is the day for you to *be* a witness. The only question is: When are you going to *do* the act of witnessing? You are now God's messenger. Go forth and share the Good News.

BREAD FOR THE SOUL

Say this prayer and write down any thoughts or requests you have for God:

Father, give me the courage to share my life's story with others. I realize that I am going to have to step out of my shell and leave my comfort zone in order for You to use me. I accept the mission that You have planned for me. I want You to use me to help others lose weight and get in shape. Father, I also pray that You would place at least one person on my path today who desperately needs to hear the Good News. Help me to make a difference in someone's life today. Amen.

_____

_____

_____

_____

_____

_____

_____

_____

_____

_____

BREAD FOR THE BODY

Perform thirty minutes of aerobic and anaerobic activity today. Ensure that your workout includes ten minutes of weight and strength training.

Day 39	Exercise Options	What I Did
30 minutes	Free weights	
	Strength training	
	Aerobics	
	Dumbbells	
	Resistance training	
	Fit for the King DVD	

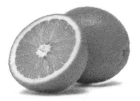

BREAD FOR THE DAY

Day 39	What to Eat	What I Ate
Breakfast 6:30–7:30 a.m.	Fast and pray	Do not eat anything
Mid-morning Snack 9:30–10:00 a.m.	Fast and pray	Do not eat anything
Lunch 12:00–1:00 p.m.	A 4-oz. tuna sandwich on wheat bread 1 Tbsp. low-fat dressing 2 celery stalks	
Mid-afternoon Snack 3:00–3:30 p.m.	6 crackers with jam 1 pear	
Dinner 5:30–8:00 p.m.	6 oz. grilled salmon 1 cup wild rice ½ cup carrots ½ cup broccoli	
Calories	**1200–1600**	

SERVING

Step 40

BREAD FOR THE MIND

God created you to complete a specific mission. He created you so He could use you to fulfill His divine purpose. No one else is qualified or capable of completing this mission but you. Your experiences, your passion, your love, and your life have all played a part in preparing you to be God's servant. The final step on this journey is to begin **serving** God. We will define *serving* as "the act of performing a task or mission for the Lord." The Great Commission is your mission. Here are some ways the Lord wants you to serve:

- **Serve to the best of your ability.**

  Each one should test his own actions. Then he can take pride in himself, without comparing himself to somebody else. (Galatians 6:4)

- **Serve to please God.**

  A person is justified by what he does and not by faith alone. (James 2:24)

- **Serve to complete your mission.**

  I consider my life worth nothing to me, if only I may finish the race and complete the task the Lord Jesus has given me. (Acts 20:24)

- **Serve like a workman.**

  Do your best to present yourself to God as one approved, a workman who does not need to be ashamed and who correctly handles the word of truth. (2 Timothy 2:15)

- **Serve like *you*.**

  There are different ways that God works through people but the same God. God works in all of us in everything we do. (1 Corinthians 12:6 NCV)

BREAD FOR THE SPIRIT

Because you are a servant of the Lord, your job is to share Jesus with as many people as possible. There is someone out there who will look at you, see the life you live, and want to know your secrets of success. You should not only deliver the message, but you must also *be* the message. You must always live your life in a manner that brings honor and glory to God. You may be the first and only Christian that some people may ever encounter. Your first impression needs to be a positive one. The way you live your life not only reflects who you are, but it also serves as a reflection on your God.

You have completed this journey, and the Lord is pleased with you. He is saying to you, *"Well done, good and faithful servant! You have been faithful with a few things; I will put you in charge of many things"* (Matthew 25:21). Today, you can go forth and prepare your heart, your mind, and your home for increase. As your reward for faithful service, the Lord has many more blessings waiting for you. Be blessed and be a blessing!

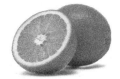

BREAD FOR THE SOUL

Say this prayer and write down any thoughts or requests you have for God:

Father, I want to thank You for bringing me to the end of this journey. I understand that this does not signify the end for me; rather, it marks the beginning of a bigger and better journey. I thank You for giving me a healthier lifestyle and a new body. I humbly accept the mission that You have planned for my life. Help me to spread Your message to others so they can also realize the size You want each of them to be. Amen.

BREAD FOR THE BODY

This is your last day! We are going to sprint the home stretch. Today, you should run for joy and run for life. Take a thirty-minute jog and remember to finish your run with a strong sprint. The finish is line is in your sights—go get it!

Day 40	Exercise Options	What I Did
30–40 minutes	Run	
	Jog	
	Power walk	

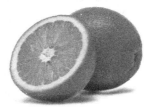

BREAD FOR THE DAY

Day 40	What to Eat	What I Ate
Breakfast 6:30–7:30 a.m.	Fast and pray	Do not eat anything
Mid-morning Snack 9:30–10:00 a.m.	Fast and pray	Do not eat anything
Lunch 12:00–1:00 p.m.	A 4-oz. turkey sandwich on wheat bread	
	1 Tbsp. low-fat dressing	
	1 cup vegetable soup	
Mid-afternoon Snack 3:00–3:30 p.m.	¼ cup almonds	
	6 strawberries	
Dinner 5:30–8:00 p.m.	6 oz. baked fish	
	1 baked potato	
	1 cup broccoli	
	2 Tbsp. salsa	
Calories	**1000–1400**	

YOUR NEW FITNESS PROFILE

Your journey is complete. It is time for you to weigh and measure your results.

You now have a forty-day journal that documents and chronicles your path to a healthier body. You can now share your personal journal with others who may struggle with weight loss or who suffer from obesity. You can also share your documented testimony with those who may desire to establish a closer relationship with God.

> *Let this be written for a future generation, that a peo ple not yet created may praise the LORD.*
>
> (Psalm 102:18)

Date: _____

Name: _____

Height: ____ ft. ____ in. Weight: ____ lbs.

Neck: _____ in. Chest: _____ in.

Waist: _____ in. Hips: _____ in.

Body fat percentage: _____
http://www.bmi-calculator.net/body-fat-calculator/

Dress or pant size: _____

Blood pressure: _____

Cholesterol level: _____

THE NEW YOU

------------Your Photo Here----------

Congratulations to the new you!

*Therefore, if anyone is in Christ, he is a new
creation; the old has gone, the new has come!*
—2 Corinthians 5:17

YOUR TESTIMONIAL

Write down your personal testimony about your experience with this book. Consider sharing it to inspire others by e-mailing it to: testimonials@fitforakingfitness.com.

Log on to our Web site at www.fitforakingfitness.com to become a member of the Fit For A King Fitness Nation. Your membership enables you to receive daily divine inspiration, motivational messages, and weekly nutritional guidance. Here you can post your comments, testimonials, and blog entries so that your story may help others.

THE FOOD EXCHANGE LIST

Since no two people are alike, this diet allows flexibility and modifications to accommodate individuals' food preferences and desires. I encourage you to be as inventive as possible in arranging meals for each day. Your creativity will keep this plan from becoming a chore.

BREAKFAST	LUNCH
ALL-BRAN	BAKED POTATO
APPLES	BLACK BEAN SOUP
BLUEBERRIES	CAESAR SALAD
CEREAL BARS	CHICKEN
CHEERIOS	COLESLAW
CORN FLAKES	CUCUMBERS
CREAM OF WHEAT	FISH
EGGS	GARDEN SALAD
ENGLISH MUFFIN	HAM SANDWICH
GRANOLA	MINESTRONE SOUP
GRITS	PASTA SALAD
KASHA CEREAL (COLD)	PB & J SANDWICH
KASHA CEREAL (HOT)	POTATO SALAD
MILK (1% or skim)	PROTEIN SHAKE
OATMEAL	ROAST BEEF
PANCAKES	SALMON
PROTEIN SHAKE	SARDINES
SHREDDED WHEAT	SCALLOPS
SOY MILK	SHRIMP
SPECIAL K CEREAL	TOMATO SOUP
TURKEY BACON	TUNA
TURKEY SAUSAGE	TURKEY
VEGETARIAN SAUSAGE	VEGETABLE SOUP
YOGURT	

THE FOOD EXCHANGE LIST

DINNER	SNACKS
ALL GREEN LEAFY VEGGIES	ALMONDS (¼ cup)
ASPARAGUS	APPLE
BAKED POTATO W/ SALSA	BANANA
BEEF TIPS	CARROT STICKS
BEETS	CASHEWS (¼ cup)
BRUSSELS SPROUTS	CELERY STALKS
BROCCOLI	CREAMSICLE
CABBAGE	DATES (¼ cup)
CHICKEN BREASTS	DILL PICKLES (2)
COLLARDS	ENGLISH MUFFIN
CUBED STEAK	FIGS (¼ cup)
GARDEN SALAD	GRANOLA BARS
GREEN BEANS	GRAPES (½ cup)
LAMB CHOPS	OLIVES (6)
MASHED POTATOES	OTHER FRUIT
MIXED VEGGIES	OTHER VEGETABLE
MUSHROOMS	PEANUT BUTTER (1 Tbsp.)
SCALLOPS	PEANUTS (½ cup)
SPINACH	PEARS
SQUASH	PINEAPPLE (½ cup)
SWEET POTATO	PLUMS
VENISON	POPCORN (2 cups)
WHITE RICE	PROTEIN BAR
WILD RICE	RAISINS (½ cup)
	RASPBERRIES
	STRAWBERRIES (6)
	STRING CHEESE

ABOUT THE AUTHOR

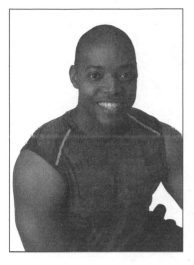

Thomas Hundley is one of the Southeast's most sought after Christian fitness and aerobics instructors. He has been leading group and personal fitness classes for more than ten years. He currently serves as the Chief of Medical Logistics in the United States Army and has attained the rank of major. He holds a Bachelor of Science degree in accounting from South Carolina State University and a Master of Science in logistics management from the Florida Institute of Technology. Thomas also holds certifications as a Group Fitness Instructor, Personal Fitness Trainer, and Sports Nutritionist.

In addition to being a published writer, Thomas is a dynamic motivational speaker who is in high demand by national Christian organizations. He is the founder and owner of Fit For a King Fitness Ministries, LLC.

Become a member of the Fit For A King Nation!
Logon to our Web site at
www.fitforakingfitness.com.
Stay connected and receive weekly nutritional guidance,
food preparation tips, and spiritual motivation.
We not only build better bodies, we build better people!

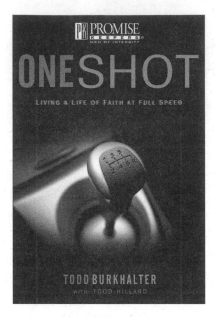

One Shot:
Living a Life of Faith at Full Speed
Todd Burkhalter

You have one shot at this life. One shot to make it count. If you
don't make the most of it, you risk wasting your life. What story
will your life tell? God designed your life to be lived with purpose,
passion, and direction. Your life was intended to mean something.
In *One Shot*, author Todd Burkhalter challenges men to live a life of
adventure and significance. True risk always begins in the heart. By
understanding who you are in Jesus Christ and who He is in you,
you can experience the adventure, meet life's challenges, and live a
significant life of faith at full speed.

ISBN: 978-1-60374-071-5 • Trade • 208 pages

WHITAKER
HOUSE

www.whitakerhouse.com